Mild Traumatic Brain Injury

Episodic Symptoms and Treatment

The first step in making any diagnosis is to think of it.
—George Thibault, M.D. (1992, p. 1664)

We see what we look for. We look for what we know.
—Johann Wolfgang von Goethe (quoted by N. D. Zasler et al., 2007, p.118)

Successful people are able to see the threads of the past and the threads of the future and untangle them into something manageable . . . the tangling is a natural state. Personalities, sunk costs, and complex systems conspire to weave the elements of our work into a matted mess. Things are the way they are, and it's difficult to perceive that they could be any other way.
—Seth Godin (2010, p. 185)

Once you know something, it's hard to imagine not knowing it.
—Chip Heath and Dan Heath (2007, p. 278)

Mild Traumatic Brain Injury

Episodic Symptoms and Treatment

Richard J. Roberts, Ph.D. and
Mary Ann Roberts, Ph.D.

In Collaboration with

Jody Murph, M.D., George C. Phillips, M.D.,
and William Sheehan, M.D.

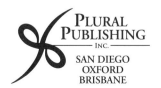

PLURAL PUBLISHING INC.

SAN DIEGO
OXFORD
BRISBANE

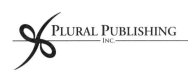

5521 Ruffin Road
San Diego, CA 92123

e-mail: info@pluralpublishing.com
Web site: http://www.pluralpublishing.com

49 Bath Street
Abingdon, Oxfordshire OX14 1EA
United Kingdom

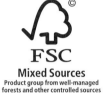

FSC
Mixed Sources
Product group from well-managed
forests and other controlled sources

Cert no. SW-COC-002283
www.fsc.org
© 1996 Forest Stewardship Council

Copyright © by Plural Publishing, Inc. 2011

Typeset in 11/14 Palatino by Flanagan's Publishing Services, Inc.
Printed in the United States of America by McNaughton and Gunn

Library of Congress Cataloging-in-Publication Data

Roberts, Richard J., 1951-
   Mild traumatic brain injury : episodic symptoms and treatment / Richard J.
Roberts and Mary Ann Roberts ; in collaboration with Jody Murph, George
Phillips, and William Sheehan.
        p. ; cm.
   Includes bibliographical references and index.
   ISBN-13: 978-1-59756-423-6 (alk. paper)
   ISBN-10: 1-59756-423-0 (alk. paper)
   1. Brain damage. I. Roberts, Mary Ann. II. Murph, Jody R. III. Phillips,
George, 1971- IV. Sheehan, William. V. Title.
   [DNLM: 1. Brain Injuries—diagnosis. 2. Brain Injuries—rehabilitation.
3. Brain Injuries—therapy. WL 354]
   RC387.5.R625 2010
   617.4'810443—dc22
                                                                    2010035147

Contents

Preface

*It's not a surprise when a scientist is surprised. That's
what happens when she is doing her job properly. To
explore, to follow hunches, to see the landscape and plot a
new course. Setting yourself up to be surprised is a
conscious choice.*

*Scientists never believe that it's all figured out,
totally settled. They understand that there's always
another argument or mystery around the corner, which
means that the map is never perfected.*

—Seth Godin (2010, p. 187)

As we move closer to publication, it has been our ultimate intention to improve care for some of the "miserable minority" of
adult and pediatric patients who sustain mild traumatic brain
injury (TBI) or brain concussion. Fortunately, the rule of thumb
is full recovery for most individuals who sustain seemingly mild
instances of head trauma. We realize that this book as a whole is
likely to represent a minority report on the state of clinical science regarding persistent mild TBI. A vocal segment of clinical
neuropsychologists contend that neurological—or brain-related
—factors seldom are primarily responsible for unexpectedly
poor outcomes among post-concussive patients; depression,
anxiety, compensation neurosis, somatizing tendencies, and factors related to litigation often are cited as the primary factors
related to poor outcome.

So-called psychological factors clearly operate in most, if not
all, cases—if only because human beings typically experience
emotional reactions when they are injured and make cognitive

attributions, both correctly and incorrectly, when they find themselves experiencing symptoms following an injury. Presently, we believe that a diverse group of patients is captured by the diagnostic criteria for Post-Concussive Syndrome or Post-Concussional Disorder. We also believe that a subgroup of this diverse group of patients experiences multiple intermittent symptoms that can significantly complicate coping with daily life. Such patients describe numerous partial seizure-like symptoms when they are interviewed systematically and comprehensively. Furthermore, the members of this subgroup respond to open trials of treatment with anticonvulsant mood stabilizers. The systematic identification of such patients is clinically crucial precisely because many such patients benefit significantly from treatment with anti-epileptic medications, even though they are not viewed as manifesting traditional forms of epilepsy.

We humbly encourage health-care professionals and interested laymen to consider our ideas, even though they may fly in the face of "the conventional wisdom." Despite conscientious efforts to provide full documentation regarding the historical bases and empirical support for our ideas, future studies of brain function and dysfunction undoubtedly will highlight the shortcomings of our presentation. As we frequently remind ourselves, "What we know now is all we know now." Mindful of our limitations, we nevertheless have persevered in writing this book as a means of ultimately influencing the assessment and clinical care of a treatable subgroup of mild TBI patients. A small, but consistent, clinical literature, ranging from the distant psychiatric writings of Emil Kraepelin to more recent studies by neurologists Dietrich Blumer and Marco Mula, has documented the existence of patients who experience multiple partial seizure-like symptoms. If we have achieved nothing else, we have compiled the majority of the relevant references from this clinical literature in a single volume.

It is possible that some experts in this field will reject our ideas out of hand without testing them out in the laboratory or the clinic. If that proves to be the case, so be it; it could not be helped. However, we believe that our work contributes a number of testable hypotheses, particularly for students and younger investigators to pursue. Furthermore, we sincerely hope that the renewed interest in mild TBI will bring some type of relief to soldiers and military veterans who have experienced blunt-force head trauma and blast exposures.

Richard J. Roberts and Mary Ann Roberts

References

Godin, S. (2010). *Linchpin.* New York, NY: Portfolio Group.

Heath, C., & Heath, D. (2007). *Made to stick.* New York, NY: Random House.

Thibault, G. (1992). Things are seldom what they seem. *New England Journal of Medicine, 327,* 1663–1666.

Zasler, N. D., Katz, D. I., & Zafonte, R. D. (2007). *Brain injury medicine: Principles and practice.* New York, NY: Demos Medical Publishing.

Acknowledgments

Foremost, we wish to acknowledge the emotional support of our family and friends.

The two primary authors wish to express gratitude to our three collaborators: Drs. Murph, Phillips, and Sheehan. We also wish to express appreciation to our many teachers and colleagues, including the late Professor Emeritus Arthur Benton and Professor Emeritus Jan Loney for challenging us to think through complex issues and to Professors John Knutson and Don Fowles of the University of Iowa for encouraging us to systematize and publish our ideas. We also wish to express appreciation to the talented individuals at Plural Publishing for their technical expertise and tolerance. A tip of the hat goes to the intrepid staff of the Hardin Medical Library of the University of Iowa. We wish to acknowledge many professional colleagues with whom we have debated many of the clinical propositions; the views of numerous supporters and critics among our professional colleagues have encouraged and challenged us to modify our ideas over the past two decades. However, any deficiencies in our presentation or controversial clinical propositions are the responsibility of the primary authors. Finally, we wish to thank our ultimate teachers—the patients we have served and their families.

Contributors

Jody R. Murph, M.D., M.S.
Associate Professor
Departments of Pediatrics and Epidemiology
Carver College of Medicine
University of Iowa
Iowa City, Iowa
Chapters 11 and 12

George C. Phillips, M.D., F.A.A.P., C.A.Q.S.M.
Clinical Associate Professor
Department of Pediatrics
Carver College of Medicine
University of Iowa
Iowa City, Iowa
Chapters 11 and 12

William Sheehan, M.D.
Psychiatric Consultant
Child and Adolescent Health Services
Wilmar, Minnesota
Medical Director
Geneva Medical Imaging
Geneva, Wisconsin
Chapters 6 and 7

This book is dedicated to the memory of our parents, Henry W. and Catherine E. Kantosky and Richard D. and Mary M. Roberts, and to the lively spirits of our younger generation: Michael, his wife Erica Finken, and our twins, Kathryn and Christopher Roberts.

Beyond the support of our relatives, we also were inspired by the efforts of the following:

- The numerous men and women who have served our nation in the Armed Forces since the inception of the global war on terror;

- Ronald Glasser, M.D., who wrote *Wounded* to call attention to the injuries and sacrifices of those who have served our nation;

- Vice President Joseph Biden, who worked as a Senator to provide additional armor for military vehicles and encouraged us to get involved;

- *USA Today* Reporter Gregg Zoroya, who somehow always manages to get the story right when it comes to covering traumatic brain injury and PTSD in OEF/OIF combat veterans;

- Admiral Michael Mullen, Chairman of the Joint Chiefs of Staff, for authorizing temporary removal from combat and additional evaluation for American troops exposed to blast concussions in Iraq and Afghanistan.

1

Brain Injury Due to Blunt-Force Trauma

*The fundamental assumption of cognitive neuroscience is
that the way we behave and the way we experience the
world is determined by the way our brains work.*
—Chris Frith (2004), *Brain*, Vol. 127, No. 2, p. 239

Introduction

The brains of human beings clearly are the products of our evo-
lutionary past (Linden, 2007). Our skulls and brains have evolved
to withstand glancing blows from rocks thrown as weapons, the
blunt force of being struck by a wooden club, or the forces resulting from minor falls. Most of the time, human brains make
robust recoveries from such instances of minor head trauma.
However, sufficient time has not passed to provide the evolu-
tionary pressure required for the skulls of human beings and the
coverings of our brains to protect us from more forceful impacts,
such as those occurring in motor vehicle crashes (Varney &
Roberts, 1999). Thus, modern life is fraught with risks to normal
brain function from so-called "blunt-force trauma."

Head trauma is a common medical cause of disrupted brain function with somewhere between 1.5 and 2 million occurrences of head trauma occurring in the United States each year (National Head Injury Foundation, 1993). Among problems treated by neurologists (i.e., physicians who specialize in diagnosing and treating diseases of the brain and nervous system), only headache ranks ahead of head trauma in terms of frequency.

The most common type of head trauma is caused by blunt-force trauma when the head strikes a fixed object (e.g., concrete pavement) or a moving object strikes the head (e.g., thrown baseball). The most common causes of head trauma in adult life include motor-vehicle accidents, falls, assaults, contact sports (e.g., football, soccer, boxing, etc.), and bicycle accidents. These types of injury are called "blunt-force" head trauma because a mechanical force is translated directly to the skull and then on to the brain. Most instances of head trauma produce either a concussion or what is sometimes called mild traumatic brain injury (TBI). Refer to Table 1–1 for the most commonly accepted definition of what constitutes a mild TBL.

At this juncture, a few words about the physical structure of the brain are in order. The brain is surrounded by three membranes that function to hold it stable inside the skull. Much like canned tuna comes packed in water or oil, the brain is encased in cerebrospinal fluid, which functions to somewhat cushion the effects of blunt-force trauma to the skull. Brain tissue itself often is described as having the consistency of firm custard. Axons, which are the long appendages of each nerve cell that lead away from the cell bodies to the dendrites of other neurons, are vulnerable to mechanical shearing and stretching from blunt-force trauma. The death of axons due to head trauma is called "diffuse axonal injury" (Li & Feng, 2009). Following trauma, there is also a "metabolic cascade" of substances in the brain, many of which may be toxic to, or alter, neuronal functioning (Giza & Hovda 2001; Werner & Engelhard, 2007). Furthermore, there is reduction in the cerebral microcirculation (Schwarzmaier, Kim, Trabold, & Plesnila, 2010). Although it was once believed that nerve cells in the brain did not regenerate after they died, recent evidence

Table 1-1. Diagnostic Criteria for Mild Traumatic Brain Injury from the American Congress of Rehabilitation Medicine (1993)

A traumatically induced physiological disruption of brain function requiring at least one of the following criteria:
• Any loss of consciousness
• Any loss of memory for events immediately before or after the accident
• Any alteration in mental state at the time of the accident (e.g., dazed)
• Focal neurologic deficit(s) that may or may not be transient
However, the severity of the injury does not exceed any of the following:
• Loss of consciousness of approximately 30 minutes or less
• After 30 minutes, an initial Glasgow Coma Scale of 13–15
• Posttraumatic amnesia not greater than 24 hours

Note: In this definition, the word "Mild" in the phrase "Mild Traumatic Brain Injury" refers only to the *acute effects* of the accident or injury and not to the long-term, clinical outcome.

Source: Adapted from: Mild Traumatic Brain Injury Committee of the Head Injury Interdisciplinary Special Interest Group (Kay et al., 1993).

suggests that some degree of neuronal regeneration is possible in selected pools of nerve cells in the brain; however, there is no guarantee that such neuronal regeneration is always *functional*— that is, neurogenesis may not necessarily lead to normalized or enhanced brain function after the brain has been injured (Ben-Ari, 2008; Hilliard, 2009).

Whereas individual neurons in the brain once were categorized as being dead or alive after blunt-force trauma to the head, recent animal research suggests that the axons of individual neurons may survive blunt-force trauma, (i.e., the neuron is still alive) but act in a dysfunctional manner due to axonal stretching (Weber, 2007). When such axonal stretching occurs in animals, alterations in the electrical mechanisms underlying synaptic transmission (i.e., how individual nerve cells communicate with one another) can result. Cells in crucial areas of the brain (such as the tissue of the hippocampus—a crucial structure in the temporal lobe for memory encoding and retrieval—and nearby areas) may become electrically unstable due to axonal stretching injuries (Cohen, Pfister, Schwarzbach, Grady, Goforth, & Satin, 2007). During most instances of blunt-force head trauma, the frontal and temporal lobes, which comprise the anterior regions of the brain, appear to be at greater risk for damage or dysfunction.

The current, conventional wisdom has been that 85% to 90% of patients who experience an instance of blunt-force head trauma will make a full recovery of function in 3 to 6 months following acute head trauma (Alexander, 1995). In the period immediately following an instance of head trauma, some patients may experience "post-concussive syndrome (PCS)" (Bigler, 2008). To make matters even more complicated, two different symptom lists for PCS exist, one adopted by the American Psychiatric Association DSM-IV-TR (American Psychiatric Association, 2000) and the other by the 10th edition *International Classification of Diseases* (World Health Organization, 1992). Both PCS lists are presented in Table 1–2. Note that these post-concussive symptoms are more or less stable from one day to the next, and that for many concussion patients or individuals with mild TBI, recovery is a gradual process.

The patients who do not recover fully within 3 to 6 months postinjury have been described by some experts as suffering from "complicated concussion" or are sometimes referred to as "the miserable minority" of patients with mild TBI (Ruff, Camenzulli, & Mueller, 1996). They also are described more formally as manifesting persistent post-concussive syndrome (PPCS) because their acute symptoms have either persisted or worsened in the 3 to 6 months following acute injury (Bigler, 2008). Unfortunately, other than antidepressant medications for those head-trauma patients who have become clinically depressed, there is a relative lack of effective treatments for patients with PPCS. In the words of experts Stein and McAllister (2009), " . . . even though tremendous progress has been made in the medical care of TBI, empirical knowledge about the management of the neuropsychi-

Table 1–2. Post-Concussive Symptoms from DMS-IV and ICD-10 Diagnostic Systems

Symptoms Common to Both Diagnostic Systems
• Dizziness
• Fatigue
• Headache
• Irritability
• Problems with memory or mental concentration
• Sleep difficulties
Additional Symptoms Unique to ICD-10
• Difficulties tolerating stress
• Emotional changes (e.g., depression, anxiety)
• Problems tolerating stress or alcohol
Additional Symptoms Unique to DSM-IV
• Changes in personality functioning (e.g., apathy, disinhibition)
• Emotional changes (other than irritability; e.g., anxiety, depression)

Note: The symptoms listed previously are not necessarily intermittent or episodic as are the symptoms of Multisymptomatic Intermittent Neurobehavioral Disorder (MIND) to be discussed later in Chapter 5.

Source: Adapted from: American Psychiatric Association. (2000). *Diagnostic and statistical manual of mental disorders* (4th ed., rev.). Washington, DC: Author; World Health Organization (1992). *International Classification of Diseases* (10th rev.).

atric sequelae of TBI is still in its infancy. This is particularly troublesome because neuropsychiatric problems are a major barrier to rehabilitation . . . " (p. 198).

What to do for a subgroup of these mild TBI patients who do not fully recover lies at the heart of this book. We propose that there is a subgroup of PPCS patients who can be described by the acronym *MIND*. MIND stands for *Multisymptomatic Intermittent Neurobehavioral Disorder*. The word "multisymptomatic" means that, when they are interviewed systematically, such patients report experiencing numerous symptoms. Patients with MIND may not complain spontaneously about all of their symptoms for a variety of reasons. Some patients, the "strong, silent types," simply try to suppress paying attention to such symptoms in order to cope with them. Other patients do not realize how frequent certain symptoms are until they are asked to specify the frequency with which each symptom occurs. Others attempt to conceal or downplay their symptoms out of concern that they may be going "crazy" or that telling the truth will have adverse impact on their careers (e.g., military rank). For these reasons, it is important that PPCS patients be given a semistructured interview (called the "Iowa Interview") by their care-providers in order to ascertain the full extent of their episodic or intermittent symptoms (Roberts, 1999).

The word "intermittent" refers to the episodic nature of many of the symptoms experienced by some PPCS patients with persistent dysfunction. The symptoms of MIND come and go (unlike the symptoms of the Post-Concussive Syndrome in Table 1–2, which typically are more static). The intermittent or episodic nature of these symptoms is a feature of MIND that troubles those care-providers who *expect* that symptoms should be constant from one time to the next in order to be valid. However, as Professor Emeritus Arthur Benton, one of the pioneers of American neuropsychology, used to lecture, "Oscillation of function is one of the hallmarks of brain damage." Similarly, Dr. Henry Head (1926), one of the giants of 20th century neurology, wrote, "An inconsistent response is one of the most striking results produced by a lesion of the cerebral cortex" (p. 145). Use of the word "intermittent" does not imply that a head-injured client *also* may not have some static or chronic problems, which are virtually always present. Both intermittent and static symptoms can co-occur following mild TBI. However, the content of the Iowa Interview was developed to study *intermittent symptoms* following head trauma (Roberts et al., 1990).

The "neuro" portion of the term "neurobehavioral" implies that the production of intermittent symptoms presumably involves the activity of the *brain* in some fashion, and the suffix "behavioral" implies that these symptoms of disrupted brain function manifest themselves in *behavior*. The most common manifestations of MIND tend to be mental (or cognitive) lapses, unexplained moods that appear to come and go for no apparent reason, brief sensory illusions, and unusual sleep phenomena.

The word "disorder" implies that the person is (a) still suffering from symptoms that interfere with daily functioning; (b) describing symptoms with statistically increased frequency as compared with healthy individuals; and/or (c) producing scores on mental tests that are unexpectedly low, despite good effort. As will be seen from the case study presented in Chapter 2, patients with symptoms of MIND tend to "fall in the cracks" between the boundaries that exist between two disciplines of academic medicine: Psychiatry and Neurology. Through no fault of their own, this state of affairs makes it difficult for patients with MIND to receive proper diagnosis and treatment. Put another way, MIND patients are neither strictly neurologic nor strictly psychiatric patients; they are neuropsychiatric patients who do not fit well within the conventional diagnostic systems for classifying primary psychiatric disorders and neurological diseases.

With regard to treatment, the major purpose of calling attention to the MIND subgroup of PPCS patients is that the functioning of MIND patients often improves with the use of a category of medications called mood-stabilizers with anticonvulsant properties (Brewerton, 1997; Monroe, 1975; Roberts, 1999). This is the major reason we believe that identifying this subtype of PPCS is so important; because the presence of MIND is likely to predict good response to a specific class of medications, even when other types of medication have been relatively ineffective. (Additional information regarding aspects of treatment follows in Chapters 6 and 7).

In summary, we are proposing that:

1. A subtype of PPCS patients manifest MIND (Multi-symptomatic Intermittent Neurobehavioral Disorder);

2. Identifying such patients is an important clinical issue, because they tend to respond well to mood-stabilizers with anticonvulsant properties;

3. Patients with MIND often go undiagnosed and untreated for extended periods of time because their clinical presentations do not fit easily into current diagnostic systems used by most neurologists and psychiatrists.

Laypersons may want to skip to Chapter 2 because the following material is relevant primarily to fellow health-care professionals, particularly those who are skeptical of evolving paradigms. In the next chapter, we discuss a composite case history to illustrate the neurobehavioral symptoms of MIND following blunt-force head trauma.

Disclaimers

We also would like to be clear with regard to what we are *not* proposing:

- We are not proposing that *all* instances of PPCS (failure to recover fully following an instance of head trauma) are due to development of the symptoms of MIND.

- We are not proposing that psychological or psychosocial factors do not exert powerful influences on clinical outcomes following head trauma.

- We are not proposing that an empirical trial of mood-stabilizing medication with anticonvulsant properties will *cure* a patient with MIND (i.e., restore a patient's function to normal or what it was prior to head trauma)— merely that many MIND patients will likely experience fewer symptoms and derive clinically significant, symptomatic relief with effective treatment.

- We are not proposing that MIND patients suffer from a traditional form of epilepsy or seizure disorder simply because they tend to respond positively to some medications whose primary use is to treat epileptic seizures.

- We are not proposing that it is impossible to malinger or exaggerate intermittent symptoms following head trauma (Wong, Regenitter, & Barrios, 1994).

- We are not proposing that *all* patients who produce high scores on the Iowa Interview necessarily suffer from MIND, in that some psychologically traumatized or highly dissociative individuals without histories of head trauma also may endorse multiple intermittent symptoms.

- We are not proposing that MIND patients also cannot have static or chronic neurobehavioral deficits (e.g., poor short-term memory, executive dysfunction), in addition to suffering from multiple intermittent symptoms.

- We are not proposing that the authors of this book have discovered a new neurobehavioral syndrome; in fact, many previous clinical neuropsychiatrists and neuropsychologists have studied and published research on this type of complex clinical entity. For the most part, we are only trying to resurrect, systematize, and illuminate the observations of the many astute clinicians and researchers who have preceded us.

- We are not proposing that blunt-force head trauma is the only cause of MIND—merely, its most common cause in industrialized societies. We also have observed the symptoms of MIND in patients with severe febrile illnesses in adulthood, other forms of thermal trauma (e.g., heatstroke), extended episodes of hypoxia (markedly reduced oxygen to the brain), and some neurotoxins.

- We are not proposing that blast-exposure injuries (such as those produced by improvised explosive devices in combat) have been proven definitively to cause symptoms of MIND; we are suggesting that this is a testable hypothesis, one that deserves additional study and research (Roberts, 2008).

■ We are not proposing that a single, comprehensive, neuropathological model fully accounts for the etiology of MIND at the present time; more experimental and clinical evidence obviously is needed to address unanswered questions.

■ We are not proposing that all care providers and clinical neuroscientists necessarily will agree with all of the concepts or hypotheses presented in this book; we are asking that our views be seriously considered, rather than having them uncritically and reflexively dismissed.

References

Alexander, M. P. (1995). Mild traumatic brain injury: Pathophysiology, natural history, and clinical management. *Neurology, 45*, 1253–1260.

American Psychiatric Association. (2000). *Diagnostic and statistical manual of mental disorders* (rev., 4th ed.). Washington, DC: Author.

Ben-Ari, Y. (2008). Epilepsies and neuronal plasticity: For better or for worse? *Dialogues in Clinical Neuroscience, 10*, 17–27.

Bigler, E. D. (2008). Neuropsychology and clinical neuroscience of persistent post-concussive syndrome. *Journal of the International Neuropsychological Society, 14*, 1–22.

Brewerton, T. D. (1997). The phenomenology of psychosis associated with complex partial seizure disorder. *Annals of Clinical Psychiatry, 9*, 31–51.

Cohen, A. S., Pfister, B. J., Schwarzbach, E., Grady, M. S., Goforth, P. B., & Satin, L. S. (2007). Injury-induced alterations in CNS electrophysiology. *Progress in Brain Research, 161*, 143–169.

Frith, C. (2004). The pathology of experience. *Brain, 127*, 239–242.

Giza, C. C., & Hovda, D. A. (2001). The neurometabolic cascade of concussion. *Journal of Athletic Training, 36*, 228–235.

Head, H. (1926). *Aphasia and kindred disorders of speech* (2 vols.). Cambridge, UK: Cambridge University Press.

Hilliard, M. A. (2009). Axonal degeneration and regeneration: A mechanistic tug-of-war. *Journal of Neurochemistry, 108*, 23–32.

Kay, T., Harrington, D. E., Adams, R., Anderson, T., Berrol, S., Cicerone, K., . . . Malec, J. (1993). *Definition of mild traumatic brain injury. Journal of Head Trauma Rehabilitation, 8*, 86–87.

Li, X. Y., & Feng, D. F. (2009). Diffuse axonal injury: Novel insights into detection and treatment. *Journal of Clinical Neuroscience, 16*, 614–619.

Linden, David. (2007). *The accidental mind*. Cambridge, MA: Harvard University Press.

Monroe, R. R. (1975). Anticonvulsants in the treatment of aggression. *The Journal of Nervous and Mental Disease, 160*, 119–126.

National Head Injury Foundation. (1993). *Interagency Head Injury Task Force reports*. Washington, DC: National Institute of Neurologic Disorders and Stroke, National Institutes of Health.

Roberts, R. J. (1999). Epilepsy Spectrum Disorder in the context of mild traumatic brain injury. In N. R. Varney & R. J. Roberts (Eds.), *The evaluation and treatment of mild traumatic brain injury* (pp. 409–447). Mahwah, NJ: Lawrence Erlbaum.

Roberts, R. J. (2008, December). Impact and the brain. *Scientific American Mind*, pp. 50–57.

Roberts, R. J., Varney, N. R., Hulbert, J. R., Paulsen, J. S., Richardson, E. D., Springer, J. A., . . . Hines, M. E. (1990). The neuropathology of everyday life: The frequency of partial seizure symptoms among normals. *Neuropsychology, 4*, 65–86.

Ruff, R. M., Camenzulli, L., Mueller, J. (1996). Miserable minority: Emotional risk factors that influence the outcome of a mild traumatic brain injury. *Brain Injury, 10*, 551–566.

Schwarzmaier, S. M., Kim, S. W., Trabold, R., & Plesnila N. (2010). Temporal profile of thrombogensis in the cerebral microcirculation after traumatic brain injury in mice. *Journal of Neurotrauma, 10*, 121–130.

Stein, M. D., & McAllister, T. W. (2009). Exploring the convergence of posttraumatic stress disorder and mild traumatic brain injury. *American Journal of Psychiatry, 166*, 768–776.

Varney, R. N., & Roberts, R .J. (1999). Forces and accelerations in car accidents and resultant brain injuries. In N. R. Varney & R. J. Roberts (Eds.), *The evaluation and treatment of mild traumatic brain injury* (pp. 39–47). Mahwah, NJ: Lawrence Erlbaum.

Weber, J. T. (2007). Experimental models of repetitive brain injuries. *Progress in Brain Research, 53*, 253–261.

Werner, C., & Engelhard, K. (2007). Pathophysiology of traumatic brain injury. *British Journal of Anaethesiology, 99*, 4–9.

Wong, J. L., Regenitter, R. P., & Barrios, F. (1994). Base rate and simulated symptoms of mild head injury among normals. *Archives of Clinical Neuropsychology, 9*, 411–425.

World Health Organization (WHO). (1992). *International classification of disease* (10th rev.). New York, NY: Author.

2

Illustrative Case History of a Patient with MIND

The pain of the mind is worse than the pain of the body.
—Publius Syrus, 1st century BC, Roman writer

In this chapter, the case history of Jane is based on a composite of three female patients. This composite reflects none of the three patients entirely due to the need to safeguard clinical confidentiality. Demographic details from these real-world cases also have been altered to ensure anonymity.

Jane was a 41-year-old professional woman who hit her head in a traffic accident roughly 13 months prior to being diagnosed and treated successfully for her multiple, episodic symptoms. Such an impact is a common form of blunt-force trauma. At the scene of the accident, she was observed to be unconscious for about 5 minutes and then to seem confused and dazed. Her first clear memory following the impact was being evaluated medically at the local emergency room. She could not recall riding in the ambulance to the hospital. An acute CT scan failed to reveal any obvious abnormalities. She was oriented adequately in the emergency room, and the medical staff decided to discharge Jane to her husband's care with instructions for him to wake her up every two to three hours to check on her during the night. The point of impact in the crash was to the left frontal area of her head, and some acute pain and bruising occurred on that side of her face, which resolved within 10 days. At the emergency room, she was prescribed a limited supply of pain medication to get her through the next few days.

Three months after the accident, Jane continued to have problems with certain post-concussive symptoms such as noise sensitivity, headache, memory lapses, difficulty sustaining attention, poor sleep, and concentration problems when working on more than one task at a time. Jane was referred to a psychiatrist by her primary care provider roughly five months following the accident because of the gradual onset of what *appeared* to be an irritable, depressive episode. Prior to the accident, Jane had been a healthy, easygoing, and well-adjusted individual. No positive family history of affective disorder existed. Litigation had not been necessary to settle insurance issues. An adequate trial of citalopram (or Celexa, an SSRI antidepressant) initiated by the psychiatrist to whom Jane was referred by her primary care-provider produced mild improvement in Jane's sleep and mood, but no improvement in her complaints of poor memory and inability to concentrate. At that point, the psychiatrist, who conscientiously had noted the history of a fairly recent instance of head trauma, referred Jane to a local neurologist for consultation.

The findings from Jane's neurological exam and an MRI scan of the structure of her brain were interpreted as being within normal limits. A standard EEG exam was read as normal, with the exception of some brief, paroxysmal theta bursts in the left temporal region of her brain, which were dismissed as a normal variant (i.e., a waveform that most likely was unrelated to her complaints).The consulting neurologist then referred Jane to a clinical neuropsychologist (a health-care professional who performs specialized testing of cognitive functioning) for a battery of mental tests. The neuropsychologist noted that Jane had above-average IQ (consistent with her strong educational and work history) and that she did indeed show problems with variable attention and concentration during formal testing. Jane's short-term memory performances also were slightly below what would be expected on the basis of her IQ, but this moderate discrepancy was attributed to her depression by the neuropsychologist. Her speed on certain timed tasks (e.g., a clerical-type coding test) also was slightly below expectations. She ultimately was diagnosed as having Persistent Post-Concussive Syndrome and Major Depressive Disorder by the neuropsychologist, and he recommended that she make special efforts to stay organized at work, maintain regular sleep habits, and consider whether or not referral to a counselor for supportive psychotherapy might be helpful.

Jane remained dissatisfied with the conservative conclusions from her neurological and neuropsychological consultations. At her next psychiatric appointment, she continued to ask whether some of her symptoms might somehow be related to the blow to the head she sustained. Her husband supported her in this and reported to the psychiatrist that he and Jane had begun to argue fairly frequently during the previous three months as to whether or not they had engaged in conversations on certain subjects. In the psychiatrist's mind, this raised the possibility of discrete memory lapses. Accordingly, the psychiatrist proposed referral to a local physiatrist (i.e., a physician specializing in rehabilitation medicine) with expertise in assessing and treating the effects of head injury in order for Jane to get a second opinion. Grudgingly, Jane agreed to yet another consultation, in large part because she felt that the only other option would have been to try a second antidepressant.

After eliciting her spontaneous complaints, the physiatrist asked Jane about the symptoms on the Iowa Interview (Roberts, 1999; Roberts et al., 1990). With regard to intermittent symptoms, Jane reported the following with an abnormally high frequency:

- Frequent illusions of a bad smell ("like burning rubber") that lasted a minute or two, but that no one else around her could smell

- Unexplained episodes of ringing in both her right and left ears for no apparent reason

- Visual illusions of movement in her right peripheral vision

- Frequent sick headaches with nausea

- Unexplained episodes of cephalic pain that were too brief to be called a headache

- Occasions when she thought the phone was ringing when it hadn't been

- Frequent word-finding lapses that had been remarked upon by her husband and co-workers

- Brief confused spells for no apparent reason

- Brief memory gaps when watching TV or movies (e.g., losing the thread of the plot)

- Unrecalled conversations (or parts of conversations) with her husband and co-workers, which she tended to insist had not occurred until confronted with undeniable evidence

- Spells of abrupt dysphoric mood that apparently were not triggered by external stimuli, even though her average mood had improved with treatment

- Spells of excessive irritability that were either not triggered or extremely out of proportion to any eliciting provocation

- Unexplained episodes of profuse nocturnal sweating, even though the bedroom was not too hot

Jane was clear that the symptoms listed previously were not always present, but would come and go unpredictably. She also reported that the onset of these intermittent symptoms was subsequent to the instance of head trauma she sustained. All other symptoms from the Iowa Interview were either endorsed with normal frequency or convincingly denied. Thus, it seemed reasonable to infer that Jane was not simply saying "Yes" to all symptoms on the interview as a cry-for-help or as a manifestation of malingering. Her total score on the Iowa Interview was well above the cut-off derived from a standardization sample of 115 healthy individuals.

Based on this information, the physiatrist referred Jane to a second neuropsychologist for a brief follow-up exam. On repeated testing, the second neuropsychologist also noted problems with attention, memory, and general slowness of processing speed; however, in addition, the second neuropsychologist administered an additional test, the Dichotic Word Listening Test (Meyers, Roberts, Bayless, Volkert, & Evitts, 2002), which challenges the patient to process two channels of auditory information simultaneously (one word to the left ear, a different word to the right ear). Despite normal hearing thresholds, Jane was impaired grossly at processing verbal information presented to her right ear, but not her left. The second neuropsychologist also tested Jane's sense of smell (something that the neurologist had failed to check) and determined that sense of smell from her left nostril was subjectively much weaker than that from her right nostril (a condition called partial *anosmia*).

Based upon these findings, the physiatrist reported back to Jane's psychiatrist his impression that Jane had indeed some persistent effects from her episode of head trauma and might benefit from a trial on a mood-stabilizing medication, such as valproic acid, in addition to her antidepressant. After some discussion between the physiatrist and the referring psychiatrist, Jane's future care was transferred to the physiatrist, and she was treated with both citalopram and valproic acid. Her abrupt episodes of depressed mood became much less frequent, as did her sensory illusions (e.g., bad odor, ringing in the ears, illusions of movement in her peripheral vision). She still was bothered occasionally by memory gaps and word-finding lapses but was able to accept practical reality-oriented counseling with regard to dealing with these residual deficits.

With Jane's permission, the Employee Assistance Program at her place of work was contacted by her physiatrist, who described the nature of her remaining difficulties and their potential impact on the job site. Some "reasonable accommodations" were implemented through Jane's supervisor and the Human Resource office at work. Coping remained difficult on a daily basis, but Jane felt considerably better off following these combined interventions. Her score on a repeated administration of the Iowa Interview had decreased significantly after six month's of care with the physiatrist. Both Jane and her husband expressed satisfaction with the long-term outcome of these interventions.

Nowhere in Jane's care did anyone make the formal diagnosis of MIND, as proposed in this book. Nor was Jane described as manifesting a traditional form of epileptic disorder. However, Jane did experience multiple, persistent symptoms from her mild TBI. Many of Jane's symptoms were *intermittent*, rather than constant or static. (For example, the ringing in her ears would come and go rather than remain constant.) There were only very subtle signs that some of her symptoms were neurobehavioral in origin: a mild EEG abnormality, inconsistent memory and attention, reduced sense of smell in one nostril, and defective dichotic processing from her right auditory channel. Considered together, Jane's constellation of symptoms can be regarded as a "disorder," in that they were statistically infrequent compared to the functioning of nonbrain-injured women of her age range and because her symptoms were causing her suffering and reduced efficiency in daily living. A seemingly mild blow to the head had disrupted the normal functioning of Jane's mind in unpredictable ways, and treatment was needed to help Jane experience fewer symptoms and accommodate to her changed life situation.

Fairly typically, Jane was treated optimally only after several different types of tests and consultations had been ordered. Her own insistence that "things had changed" following an instance of minor head trauma, the support of her husband, and the flexibility and diligence of her consulting psychiatrist were all factors that contributed to her positive clinical outcome. Although Jane's life had been altered substantially by a single instance of mild TBI, this case study represents a positive clinical outcome.

In the next chapter, we review why it can be quite difficult for brain-injured individuals with PPCS and symptoms of MIND following head trauma to find appropriate diagnosis and optimal treatment in today's health-care system.

References

Englot, D. J. (2009). *Partial seizures and consciousness: Insight from rodent models*. New Haven, CT: Create Space.

Meyers, J. E., Roberts, R. J., Bayless, J. D., Volkert, K., & Evitts, P. E. (2002). Dichotic listening: Expanded norms and clinical application. *Archives of Clinical Neuropsychology*, *17*, 79–90.

Roberts, R. J. (1999). Epilepsy Spectrum Disorder in the context of mild traumatic brain injury. In N. R. Varney & R. J. Roberts (Eds.), *The evaluation and treatment of mild traumatic brain injury* (pp. 209–447). Mahwah, NJ: Lawrence Erlbaum.

Roberts, R. J., Varney, N. R., Hulbert, J. R., Paulsen, J. S., Richardson, E. D., Springer, J. A., . . . Hines, M. E. (1990). The neuropathology of everyday life: The frequency of partial seizure symptoms among normals. *Neuropsychology*, *4*, 65–86.

3

Navigating the Health-Care System Following Mild TBI

When we don't even believe that something is possible or that it exists, we fail to see it at all.
—Dorothy Otnow Lewis, American psychiatrist,
Guilty by Reason of Insanity (1998, pp. 615–616)

For the composite case study in the previous chapter, let's review the number of different health-care providers with whom Jane had contact:

- Paramedics at the scene of the accident
- ER physicians and staff
- CT scan techs and radiologist
- Her primary care provider who referred Jane to the Psychiatrist
- The neurologist and his staff

- The EEG tech who performed the EEG (brain-wave) test

- A different neurologist who interpreted her EEG

- The first clinical neuropsychologist and his testing technician

- The physiatrist (rehabilitation medicine physician) and his staff

- The second clinical neuropsychologist

In this era of increasing medical and technological specialization, it is apparent that a single blow to the head can lead to numerous interactions with health-care professionals and can generate substantial medical bills for diagnostic studies when symptoms persist. With considerable perseverance on Jane's part, the contributions of multiple health-care specialists eventually were sufficient to develop a coherent and successful strategy for Jane's treatment, one that permitted her to remain gainfully employed. However, such positive outcomes following persistent mild TBI are not always the rule.

Previous research studies have documented that the individuals with brain injuries have significant, unmet, medical needs in the American health-care system (e.g., Heinemann, Sokol, Gavin, & Bode, 2002; Slomine et al., 2006; Pickelsimer et al., 2007). As a result, patients who suffer from the subtle effects of brain dysfunction following head trauma can go months, or even years, without accurate diagnosis and adequate treatment. Gordon and colleagues have termed such outcomes "hidden" cases of traumatic brain injury (Gordon et al., 1998). Associations between traumatic brain injury and important social problems, such as drug use, domestic abuse, unemployment, homelessness, crime, delinquency in minors, and increased risk of suicide, have been documented repeatedly in published research.

So why do many patients with mild TBI, PPCS, and MIND miss getting properly diagnosed and treated? Several main reasons exist for this state of affairs.

First and foremost, *there currently is no well-accepted, single diagnostic category for patients with MIND* in the classification systems developed by academic psychiatry and neurology to describe major categories of psychiatric disorder and neurologic disease. Although mentioned in the first chapter of this book, this observation bears repeating. In the words of Thibault (1992), "The first step in making any diagnosis is to think of it." Unfortunately, the lack of a single, agreed-upon, diagnostic label prevents MIND patients from being recognized, even after the diagnosis of PPCS has been made. Furthermore, making the diagnosis of PPCS does not always lead to optimal treatment with medications; this is because most clinicians do not assess for intermittent symptoms with the Iowa Interview. Additionally, well-respected experts have cautioned that treating dysfunctional PPCS patients with medications is to be avoided lest the care provider unwittingly reinforce the sick role—thereby leading to a future of constant doctor shopping and avoidance of facing psychological or psychiatric factors that sustain dysfunction in daily life (e.g., Alexander, 1995).

Practically speaking, care providers look for the diagnoses and symptoms that they have been trained to look for during their formal training. As mentioned previously, MIND following blunt-force trauma is a neuropsychiatric syndrome, one that is neither solely the concern of neurology or psychiatry. A key reason why we chose to promote the acronym MIND to describe this loosely defined syndrome is because MIND is memorable (Heath & Heath, 2007). Hopefully, this mnemonic may prompt more physicians and care providers to interview for the types of fleeting or spell-like, intermittent symptoms that can arise following mild TBI.

The remainder of this chapter focuses on less salient reasons why patients like Jane often seem to have difficulty getting the professional help they need.

1. *The odds are with full recovery.* For every patient like Jane who continues to have significant problems following

mild TBI, probably eight or nine patients appear to recover fully by 3 to 6 months postaccident. Therefore, if patients are provided supportive medical care in the acute phase of injury, psycho-educational materials about the natural course of mild TBI, encouraged to rest, do not need to get involved in protracted litigation, and manage to avoid any subsequent instances of head trauma, the odds are that most of them will recover. Thus, after initial evaluation, conservative care —or "watchful waiting," as it sometimes is called— often is viewed as an appropriate approach to management, unless complications are apparent immediately. Jane continued to be dissatisfied with her clinical outcome when she did not recover to her preinjury level of functioning.

2. *The misleading semantics of TBI suggest that "mild" impacts are unlikely to have serious and persistent effects.* The "mild" in "mild TBI" refers only to the *acute effects* of blunt-force impact on the brain—and *not* to the longer term, clinical outcome of the patient who sustains an instance of blunt-force impact. This is one of the few times in all of clinical medicine when a disease or a condition is rated as mild based upon the acute outcome (e.g., brief loss of consciousness) rather than the longer term impact on the patient's functioning. Thus, it is entirely possible to sustain a mild TBI and yet experience clinically significant problems (as Jane did), and it also is possible to experience a moderately severe TBI but excellent longer term recovery with few, if any, residual problems (Roberts, 2008).

3. *The care-provider fails to obtain (or the patient fails to provide) a history of past TBI.* Sometimes health-care providers and behavioral practitioners fail to ask about a history of head trauma, especially if no trauma history has been documented previously in a given patient's medical records. Also, primary care providers may not

inquire regarding previous head injury if the patient's primary complaints and symptoms appear to be unrelated to head trauma. To remedy this state of affairs, some head trauma experts are developing instruments to encourage patients to disclose past instances of head trauma.

When interviewing patients, it is helpful to ask about history of possible head trauma in a variety of different ways:

- Have you ever been knocked out?
- Have you ever lost consciousness due to a blow to the head?
- Have you ever been in a motor vehicle accident?
- Have you ever cracked a windshield with your head?
- Have you ever been assaulted or hit in the head?
- Have you ever had any near-death experiences?

Although these questions may seem redundant, it is not uncommon for the third or fourth query in such a series of questions to prompt the retrieval of pertinent information regarding a history of head trauma. Thus, even though a care provider asks specifically about head trauma, the patient may fail to describe one or more instances of it.

Problems with recall of episodic events are frequent following TBI, and some patients simply may fail to recall a clear instance of head trauma. Also, if there has been a gradual onset of problems following head trauma, patients (and care providers) may fail to make a connection between the initiating event and the subsequent emergence of symptoms (Roberts, 1999).

The first author has observed more than one patient initially deny a history of head trauma, only to have the same patient come back days later and report a potentially significant instance of head impact after pondering the question or consulting relatives. In such instances, the clinician who takes the second history (or even third) is often the "hero." For these reasons, it can be helpful if the patient is interviewed in the presence of a parent, spouse, significant other, or close friend—a collateral informant who may be in a position to supplement or correct a patient's faulty or inefficient recall.

4. *Some clinicians and experts act as though they believe that the presence of litigation can explain completely why some patients have persistent symptoms.* If you are injured in a motor vehicle accident, and you are not at fault, you unfortunately may need to sue the driver of the vehicle that hit you (or their insurance carrier) in order to recover medical costs and other damages. Apparently, some clinicians who spend a good deal of their practice working as forensic witnesses in civil litigation have become convinced that the presence of ongoing litigation inevitably explains the severity and persistence of the patient's symptoms and complaints following mild TBI. If this type of skepticism or bias goes unchecked, it can lead a practitioner to misattribute subtle problems to psychological factors that may well be due subtle brain dysfunction following head injury (Persinger, 2000; Ruff, 2009). (For those professionals who derive substantial income from forensic practices, it may be important to accept referrals from both defense attorneys and plaintiffs' attorneys to avoid any unspoken expectations to deliver a biased impression favorable to one side or the other. At the outset of conversation with a litigant's attorney, it also can be important to insist that, if the litigant suffers from a potentially treatable syndrome such as MIND, the evaluating expert retains the right to refer the litigant for possible treatment, if warranted.)

In the interest of full disclosure, neither of the two primary authors of this book actively engages in forensic practice.

5. *Some practitioners believe that psychological factors are far more important than physiological or brain-related factors in determining which patients go on to manifest PPCS.* This excerpt from Dr. Michael P. Alexander's influential 1995 clinical review of mild traumatic brain injury is fairly typical of this conservative perspective:

> Management of PPCS [Persistent Post-Concussive Syndrome] is a mixture of somatic treatments, psychological-psychiatric management and pragmatic occupational interventions. Patients, and usually their families, will not believe that the disability is not caused by brain injury in a perfectly straightforward cause and effect way. . . . Care must be taken that they don't find a therapist who assumes that their symptoms all represent real neurologic loss. (p. 1258–1259)

A recent review of the issue of persistent dysfunction following blunt-force "mild" TBI by neuropsychiatrists Jonathan Silver, Robert Hales, and Stuart Yudofsky in 2008 takes a somewhat more moderate stance:

> The majority of individuals with mild TBI recover quickly, with significant and progressive reduction in all three [symptom] domains (cognitive, somatic, and behavioral) at 1, 3, and certainly 6 months from the injury . . . Unfortunately, good recovery is not universal. A significant number of patients continue to complain of persistent difficulties 6–12 months and even longer after their injury . . . Therefore, there may be two groups of mild TBI patients: those who recover by 3 months and those who have persistent symptoms. It is not known whether the persistent symptoms are part of a cohesive syndrome or simply represent a collection of loosely related symptoms resulting from the vagaries of an individual

injury. However, it is increasingly recognized that 'mild' TBI and concussions that occur in sports injuries result in clinically significant neuropsychological impairment." (pp. 615–616)

This more balanced view echoes the opinion of Ryan and Warden in their 2003 review of the literature on post-concussive syndrome:

Most investigators now believe that a variety of pre-morbid, injury-related, and post-morbid neuropathological and psychological factors contribute to the development and continuation of these symptoms in those sustaining mild traumatic brain injury (MTBI). (p. 310)

A care provider or expert who believes that psychological factors are almost always more crucial than brain-related factors in sustaining the effects of a seemingly minor instance of head trauma is less likely to search for symptoms of MIND—and more likely to attribute such symptoms to emotional causes, such as a tendency to engage in somatization (Lamberty, 2007) or hypochondriasis (Boone, 2009). Thus, the intermittent symptoms and complaints of patients with MIND ultimately may be dismissed as "medically unexplained physical symptoms"—ones that do not require further medical investigation or intervention (Allanson, Bass, & Wade, 2002; Carson et al., 2003; Creed, 2009)

6. *Some practitioners are concerned that focusing on attempts to treat the patient's symptoms too quickly or too aggressively will end up turning transient post-concussive symptoms into hardened PPCS.* In this regard, Wood (2007) has cautioned, "Patients' perceptions of their illness early after head injury may play a part in the persistence of post-concussional syndrome" (p. 552). Similarly, with regard to diagnosis and management of possible mild brain injuries from combat, Bryant (2008) recommended:

> . . . soldiers should not be led to believe that hav-
> ing a brain injury will result in permanent
> change. . . . If troops currently serving in Iraq or
> Afghanistan are informed about a postconcus-
> sive syndrome and persistent problems emerg-
> ing from mild traumatic brain injury, a new
> syndrome could arise from the current conflict
> in which soldiers attribute a range of common
> stress reactions to the effects of brain injury. This
> could be damaging to morale and to the per-
> son's future mental health, because it could lead
> to the expectation of poor recovery. In contrast,
> the normalization of many of these reactions and
> the recognition that stress-related conditions can
> be managed with evidence-based strategies may
> minimize the unnecessary attribution of common
> stress reactions to pathology and facilitate resil-
> ience after mild traumatic brain injury. (p. 526)

Thus, some clinicians may be reticent to ask detailed
questions (such as those in the Iowa Interview) following
mild head trauma lest they be accused by more conservative colleagues of planting the seeds of iatrogenic
(i.e., doctor-caused) illness in the minds of patients.

7. *If subjective symptoms are important following mild TBI,
then the patient should be expected to describe them during
an open-ended interview in a coherent fashion.* During an
open-ended interview (i.e., one in which the patient
describes in a general and unprompted way the symptoms and complaints of concern), most patients with
MIND describe the sorts of *trait-like* post-concussive
symptoms listed in Table 1–2. However, the intermittent symptoms of MIND are much more *state-like* or
fleeting, in that they come and go unpredictably and
may last only a few seconds or minutes at a time. This
is one reason why we recommend that care providers
spend the time to administer a semistructured interview,

such as the Iowa Interview, to assess episodic symptoms in a systematic fashion. Although taking a detailed history does require valuable clinical time early on, it is generally better to be thorough at the beginning of a brain injury evaluation than to overlook potentially important symptoms.

When interviewing an individual with brain injury, the clinician frequently needs to reorganize aspects of information provided by the patient. For this reason, it is helpful to have a standard interview format such as the Iowa Interview to help both the clinician and patient stay on track. (A patient's inability to provide a coherent history on first telling may raise suspicion on the part of skeptical clinicians regarding the legitimacy of the patient's presentation.) Patients who sustain damage or dysfunction to the prefrontal regions of the brain can have difficulties with providing an accurate chronology of events, may misinterpret the meaning of individual questions, or have difficulty providing frequency estimates of certain symptoms. (As mentioned previously, it is also helpful for the interviewer to have access to collateral informants with extensive knowledge of the patient's history and recent functioning.)

8. *There is a relative lack of research on the effects of many types of medications in treating mild TBI and MIND.* Therefore, until formal research on treatment outcome substantiates or refutes the clinical recommendations of experts, promising case studies, and the results of open-trials of medications, more skeptical or conservative physicians may be understandably reluctant to consider treating a subgroup of patients, such as MIND patients, because mood-stabilizers with anticonvulsant properties occasionally can have serious side effects. (The ramifications of this issue are discussed in more detail in Chapter 6 and Chapter 7 dealing with treatment with medication.)

9. *Given our national issues with the use of illicit drugs, a back-lash has occurred on the part of some segments of the patient population (e.g., military, people who work in law enforcement, politically conservative individuals, and some elderly individuals) against "Big Pharma" and the use of prescription medications to treat problems that appear to be, in part, behavioral or psychological (e.g., rapid mood swings).* A major purpose of making a clinical diagnosis is that doing so will lead to an effective plan of treatment. In an understudied area, such as the pharmacological treatment of mild TBI, a significant minority of patients may resist the prospect of treatment with medications for personal reasons. Patients may object that "medication is a crutch" or that "real men don't take pills." In such instances, the patient obviously has the "final vote." Leaving the option of possible treatment open (should the patient change his or her mind in the future) and parting amicably sometimes is necessary on the part of the care provider.

10. *Lack of insurance coverage or lack of access to specialty care may prevent some patients from receiving necessary services.* As this chapter was being written, heated debate raged over the need for health-care reform in the United States. In addition to specialty care from neurologists and psychiatrists, patients with MIND may need to consult subspecialists, such as neuropsychiatrists, behavioral neurologists, and neuropsychologists, in order to clarify diagnostic issues. Unfortunately, unrecognized or under-treated symptoms following mild TBI may be associated with declining vocational status, reduction in personal wealth, and limited access to broad medical coverage.

Summary

In summary, the lack of a single, agreed-upon, diagnostic term for MIND has undoubtedly been the major reason for this proposed subgroup of PPCS patients having been overlooked by health-care professionals. However, numerous other factors having to do with our health-care system, prescribing tendencies of individual providers, and current clinical practices also have helped complicate access to care, proper diagnosis, and effective treatment for such patients.

The next chapter will review previous clinical and research evidence that supports the existence of MIND as a syndrome and its association with blunt-force head trauma. In this regard, the following chapter may be of greater interest or relevance to health-care practitioners and/or clinical researchers than to TBI patients themselves. The material to be discussed may be perceived by some lay readers as excessively detailed or technical. However, we have tried to present evidence for the existence of MIND due to blunt-force trauma in a straightforward manner that will be accessible to interested lay readers, particularly those with some background in health care or behavioral research.

References

Alexander, M. P. (1995). Mild traumatic brain injury: Pathophysiology, natural history, and clinical management. *Neurology, 45*, 1253–1260.

Allanson J., Bass, C., Wade, D. T. (2002). Characteristics of patients with persistent severe disability and medically unexplained neurological symptoms: A pilot study. *Journal of Neurology, Neurosurgery, and Psychiatry, 73*, 307–309.

Boone, K. B. (2009). Fixed belief in cognitive dysfunction despite normal neuropsychological scores: Neurocognitive hypochondriasis? *Clinical Neuropsychologist, 23*, 1016–1036.

Bryant, R. A. (2008). Disentangling mild traumatic brain injury and stress reactions. *New England Journal of Medicine, 358*, 525–527.

Carson, A. J., Best, S., Postma, K., Stone J., Warlow, C., & Sharpe, M. (2003). The outcome of neurology outpatients with medically unexplained symptoms: A prospective cohort study. *Journal of Neurology, Neurosurgery, and Psychiatry, 74*, 897–900.

Creed, F. (2009). The outcome of medically unexplained symptoms—will DSM-V improve on DSM-IV somatoform disorders? *Journal of Psychosomatic Research, 66,* 379–381.

Gordon, W. A., Brown, M., Sliwinski, M., Hibbard, M. R., Patti, N., Weiss, M. J., . . . Sheerer, M. (1998). The enigma of "hidden" traumatic brain injury. *Journal of Head Trauma Rehabilitation, 13,* 39–56.

Heath, C., & Heath, D. (2007). *Made to stick: Why some ideas die and others survive.* New York, NY: Random House.

Heinemann, A. W., Sokol, K., Garvin, L., & Bode, R. K. (2002). Measuring unmet needs and services among persons with traumatic brain injury. *Archives of Physical Medicine and Rehabilitation, 83,* 1052–1059.

Lamberty, G. J., (2007). *Understanding somatization in the practice of clinical neuropsychology.* New York, NY: Oxford University Press.

Lewis, D. L. (1998). *Guilty by reason of insanity.* New York, NY: Ivy Press.

Persinger, M. A. (2000). Subjective improvement following treatment with carbamazepine (Tegretol) for a subpopulation of patients with traumatic brain injuries. *Perceptual and Motor Skills, 90,* 37–40.

Pickelsimer, E. E., Selassie, A. W., Sample, P. L., Heinemann, A. W., Gu, J. K., & Veldheer, L. C. (2007). Unmet service needs of persons with traumatic brain injury. *Journal of Head Trauma Rehabilitation, 22,* 1–13.

Roberts, R. J. Epilepsy Spectrum Disorder in the context of mild traumatic brain injury. (1999). In N. R. Varney & R. J. Roberts (Eds.), *The evaluation and treatment of mild traumatic brain injury* (pp. 209–447). Mahwah, NJ: Lawrence Erlbaum.

Roberts, R. J. (December, 2008). Impact and the brain. *Scientific American Mind,* pp. 50–57.

Ruff, R. (2009). Best practice guidelines for forensic neuropsychological examinations with traumatic brain injury. *Journal of Head Trauma Rehabilitation, 24,* 131–140.

Ryan, L. M., & Warden, D. L. (2003). Post concussion syndrome. *International Review of Psychiatry, 15,* 310–316.

Silver, J. M., Hales, R. E., & Yudofsky, S. C. (2002). Neuropsychiatric aspects of traumatic brain injury. In Yudofsky, S. C. & Hales, R. E. (Eds.), *The American Psychiatric Publishing Textbook of Neuropsychiatry and Behavioral Neursosciences* (pp. 595–647). New York, NY: American Psychiatric Association.

Slomine, B. S., McCarthy, M. L., Ding R., MacKenzie, E. J., Jaffe, K. M., Durbin, D. R., . . . Paidas, C. N. (2006). Health care utilization and needs after pediatric traumatic brain injury. *Pediatrics, 117*, e663–674.

Thibault, G. E. (1992). Things are seldom what they seem. *New England Journal of Medicine, 327*, 1663–1666.

Wood, R. L. (2007). "Post concessional" syndrome: All in the minds eye! *Journal of Neurology, Neurosurgery, and Psychiatry, 78*, 552.

4

Evidence for the Existence of MIND-like Neuropsychiatric Patients

The farther backward you look, the farther forward you are likely to see.

—Winston Churchill

Support From the Neuropsychiatric Literature

Patients similar to those we have labeled as manifesting MIND have been described repeatedly in the modern, neuropsychiatric literature. (A neuropsychiatrist is a physician with extensive training in both psychiatry and neurology and is, thus, in an excellent position to assess and treat patients who fall in the "boundary lands" between the two disciplines.)

Perhaps the most succinct description of such patients was provided by neuropsychiatrist Michael Alan Taylor in his 1999 text, *Fundamentals of Clinical Neuropsychiatry*:

[These] patients typically complain of persistent dysphoria. They have angry, sometimes violent outbursts that fill
them with remorse and sometimes lead to suicide. They
are more likely to damage furniture or themselves than
other persons. They are more concerned about "going
crazy," may hallucinate, and develop a positive symptom psychosis. They complain of illusions of peripheral
movement, tinnitus, word-finding problems, speaking
jargon, "confusional spells," (brief and usually unnoticed
by others), memory gaps, unrecalled behavior, staring,
depressive and anxiety spells, and angry outbursts. . . .
Consider epilepsy spectrum disorder when a patient
has persistent dysphoria and multiple complex partial
seizure-like symptoms but no stereotyped spells or
motor automatisms. Whether these patients are, in fact,
epileptics with a deep brain focus or have another tem-
porolimbic disorder is unknown, but they respond to
anticonvulsants." (p. 307)

The syndrome described by Taylor as "epilepsy spectrum disorder" basically is quite comparable to the concept of MIND, as
presented in this book. However, the present authors have chosen the neutral acronym, MIND, over epilepsy spectrum disorder in the hope of avoiding fruitless controversy over whether
such patients are truly epileptic or not (Crompton & Berkovic,
2009). We have found that such debate tends to be unproductive
and actually distracts health-care providers from considering the
proposition that such poly-symptomatic patients actually exist
and are in need of treatment. For Taylor, the key features of the
syndrome appeared to be (a) frequent, untriggered mood-swings;
(b) sensory illusions and unformed hallucinations; and (c)
episodic or intermittent cognitive lapses. Taylor noted that such
patients responded favorably to treatment with anticonvulsant
mood stabilizers and implied that the anterior (e.g., temporolim-
bic) portions of the brain likely were involved. Taylor did not
implicate blunt-force head injury as the major cause of the syn-

drome, but clearly implied that the brains of such patients likely were be damaged or dysfunctional in some fashion.

Some 13 years earlier, neuropsychiatrist Gary Tucker had published a series of 20 cases with clinical presentations that corresponded closely to the profile later described by Taylor in 1999. According to Tucker and his colleagues (Tucker, Price, Johnson, & McAllister, 1986), the major features of their patients were as follows:

- Multiple "spells" and episodic symptoms that appear to come and go for no apparent reason

- Intense, untriggered mood swings

- Brief memory lapses, confusional spells, and word-finding spells

- Episodic sensory illusions or unformed hallucinations

- Chronic unhappiness (i.e., persistent dysphoria), with frequent suicidal ideation and attempts

- Unusual nocturnal phenomena, such as sleep-talking, parasomnias, and repetitive nightmares

Tucker and his associates observed that most of their patients responded well to anticonvulsant medications, even though they previously had exhibited poor clinical response to antidepressants, antipsychotics, and lithium (all of which lowered seizure threshold to some extent). Although their EEG results were typically "abnormal" in some way, these brain-wave tests were not clearly diagnostic of most conventional seizure disorders. Tucker noted that the patients in his case series were "typical neither of most psychiatric patients nor of most patients with seizure disorder" (p. 348). Furthermore, Tucker found that these patients had been frequently misdiagnosed:

Virtually all of the patients had been initially and often multiply [mis]diagnosed as having primary psychiatric disturbances of a functional type even though very few met DSM-III diagnostic criteria. . . . Careful diagnostic evaluation is of obvious importance in patients such as these in whom drug treatment is both indicated and likely to provide benefit with respect to the behavioral pathology in question. (p. 356)

When such patients were not suffering discrete spells (e.g., bouts of rage), social behavior relatively was normal, and cognitive functioning often was unremarkable on mental status examination. Their transient or episodic problems with thinking and remembering were similar to those experienced by some epileptic individuals between frank seizures. Tucker's research team did not link this clinical presentation specifically to the effects of head trauma. Nor did they speculate on other causes for this loosely defined syndrome. During a conversation with the first author of this book, the now deceased Professor Emeritus Tucker related that there was at first considerable resistance on the part of journal reviewers to considering his manuscript in a favorable light (Tucker, personal communication, 1993).

Some 21 years prior to the publication of Tucker's paper, a psychiatrist named A.D. Jonas (1965) published a book titled, *Ictal and Subictal Neurosis*, in which he described a series of polysymptomatic patients similar to those later described by Taylor and Tucker. Apparently, Jonas first developed a research interest in such patients from observing the neurobehavioral changes in the son of a close friend after the boy reportedly sustained brief loss of consciousness during a collision in a basketball game. Although relatively few effective anticonvulsant medications were available during that time, the majority of the patients in Jonas's series responded favorably to treatment with phenytoin (Dilantin), even though they had responded poorly on other types of psychiatric medications. Jonas emphasized that the patients in his case series were rather skeptical that any pharmacological treatment would provide symptomatic relief:

From the beginning, most of these patients were essentially distrustful and required considerable persuasion

before accepting any medication. Their prevailing atti-
tude was pessimistic and hopeless, as if they did not
believe anything could help them . . . (p. vii)

In a brief note in the *American Journal of Psychiatry* in 1977,
Dr. Jonas expressed discouragement that neurologists and psychiatrists still had great difficulty identifying such "borderland"
patients as being in need of treatment. He also expressed his
opinion that head trauma might well have something to do with
the difficulties of his poly-symptomatic patients:

> Beyond the theoretical interest of this phenomenon is a
> clinically important consideration. As a psychiatrist in an
> Army hospital, I see many young men who are brought
> in as a result of a violent or antisocial outburst. In a sur-
> prisingly large proportion of these instances, even a brief
> interview discloses a history of head injuries after which
> these men notice a change in behavior for which they
> cannot offer any explanation; in some cases there is a time
> lapse between the injury and such cases. . . . It requires a
> major reorientation to the thinking of both neurologists
> and psychiatrists to acknowledge the existence of this
> wide borderland. (p. 1052)

With regard to the lack of routinely abnormal brain-wave
tests on standard EEG exams, Jonas asserted:

> Neurologists consistently deny the existence of the con-
> dition unless textbook symptoms are accompanied by
> abnormal EEGs. However, somewhere along the gradient
> of illness, CNS events that are not severe enough to pro-
> duce EEG changes are still capable of producing symptoms
> of spontaneous cerebral discharges. (p. 1051)

Jonas went on to praise the emerging work of neuropsychiatrist Dorothy Otnow Lewis, who had begun to publish data indicating that violent delinquents frequently experienced multiple

intermittent symptoms in the context of histories of pre-existing head trauma. Later in her career, Dr. Lewis, along with neurologist Jonathan Pincus (Lewis & Pincus, 1989), reported that severely violent delinquents, including 14 murderers on death row, frequently reported experiencing multiple partial seizure-like symptoms (i.e., similar to the intermittent or episodic symptoms of MIND). According to Lewis and Pincus (1989), this clinical feature, when combined with cruelty and paranoid ideation, was associated with a propensity for episodic violence and rage outbursts.

Shortly after the publication of Jonas's monograph (1965), an article authored by a European clinician named Smoczynski (1972) independently identified a "temporal lobe syndrome" in patients with epilepsy characterized by sudden mood swings and other episodic symptoms. This temporal lobe syndrome appeared to be independent of the patients' seizure disorders and occurred in 32% of cases studied between 1961 and 1969 at the Gdansk Medical Academy. In the author's own words:

> The patients complained that they could not make a proper use of their previously achieved experiences and knowledge despite preservation of a relatively high level of basic intellectual functions. The activities of patients often were governed by the state of their mood at a given moment; they had the character of the so-called "short-circuits" caused by sudden mood swings. (p. 1713)

Smoczynski also referenced the 20th century European, epileptologist Landolt, as having made similar observations. (Note that Blumer (2000), an American epileptologist, has documented that features of "interictal dysphoric disorder" or "temporal lobe syndrome" can be traced back to the writings of Kraepelin and Bleuler, two of the European forefathers of modern biological psychiatry.) Smoczynski observed that most patients with temporal lobe syndrome (in addition to the seizure disorder) did not manifest clear deficits on formal cognitive testing, "Clinical psychological testing failed to demonstrate any gross abnormalities of intellectual function" (p. 1711). The most common etiology for seizures in his patients was described as "skull trauma" (i.e., blunt-force impact to the head).

Hayes and Goldsmith (1991) studied the clinical features of affectively ill psychiatric patients who responded positively to two anticonvulsant mood stabilizers, valproic acid and carbamazepine. They found that patients who responded favorably to these mood stabilizers tended to endorse significantly more intermittent symptoms than patients who responded to traditional psychotropic medications, such as antidepressants and lithium. In their words:

> A perusal of the data, then, suggests that alterations in the sensory pathways (altered sound quality, unformed auditory hallucinations, olfactory hallucinations, altered odor intensity, altered light intensity, altered distance, taste hallucinations, and tactile distortions) rapidity of mood change, (sudden depression, sudden rage, sudden dysphoria) and disturbances in the flow of thought (speeded thoughts, slowed thoughts, jumbled thoughts), along with speech arrest, jamais vu, and time disorientation were associated with a positive response to anticonvulsants compared to a population of equal size of responders to standard psychopharmacological agents. Furthermore, sensory function disturbance . . . and rapidity of mood change (sudden depression, sudden rage), along with amnestic episodes [memory gaps] and speech arrest, were significantly more common in pure anticonvulsant responders when compared to a group of lithium responders of approximately equal size. (pp. 32–33)

Furthermore, Hayes and Goldsmith proposed a spectrum concept, in which there likely was to be a "borderland territory with gradations, between overt temporal lobe epilepsy [i.e., partial seizure disorder] and pure affective disorder" (p. 33). Findings from subsequent survey studies with unselected subjects have supported their concept of a continuum of neuro-electric stability ranging from few, in any, intermittent symptoms endorsed to the experiencing of multiple intermittent symptoms (Persinger & Makarec, 1993; Ryan et al., 2006).

Then in 1992, a relatively obscure, nonacademic physician (who treated many individuals with mild-to-moderate blunt-force TBI), Walter Verduyn, noted that a number of his patients who failed to recover fully from mild-to-moderate TBI suffered from the symptoms similar to those described by Tucker et al. (Verduyn, Hilt, Roberts, & Roberts, 1992). Most of the patients in Verduyn's case series also benefited from open trials of treatment with anticonvulsant medications, even though they had not improved following treatment with other types of medications. Verduyn and his associates suggested that such patients likely suffered from subclinical electrical instability that was caused by one or more instances of blunt-force head trauma. Put another way, it seemed possible that such patients had developed electrically unstable brains—but not necessarily traditional epilepsy.

In 1996, neurologist Marc Hines and his associates, who were familiar with both Tucker's and Verduyn's studies, proposed an anatomical model to explain how the clinical syndrome of epilepsy spectrum disorder might occur (Hines, Swan, Roberts, & Varney, 1995). Hines reasoned that damage to relatively few brain cells in crucial locations involving portions of a small structure in the temporal lobes called the hippocampal region theoretically could produce the sort of poly-symptomatic clinical picture previously described by Jonas, Tucker, and Verduyn, among others.

More recently, a team of Norwegian investigators has identified a subgroup of depressed patients whom they refer to as suffering from "Acute Unstable Depressive Syndrome" (AUDS). Such patients are characterized by "brief depressive episodes" in the context of "rapidly fluctuating psychiatric symptoms" and reportedly do not fit well into with any current diagnostic criteria (Bjork et al., 2008). In addition to brief periods of dysphoric mood, such patients manifested explosive irritability, delusions, confusion, and anxiety symptoms. When compared with a group of patients with uncomplicated depressions, AUDS patients showed multiple abnormal features in their standard EEG exams, but did not show an increase in clearly epileptiform activity. When quantitative EEG (a sophisticated type of computerized brain-wave analysis) was used to study cerebral electrical activity, additional significant differences were observed between the two groups. The authors reasoned that, "Organic brain dysfunction may be involved in the pathogenesis of patients with brief depressive episodes mixed with rapidly fluctuating psychiatric symptoms" (p. 1).

In a follow-up study from the same team of investigators (Vaaler et al., 2009), a sample of AUDS patients had significantly more conventional seizures in their clinical histories and a significantly higher frequency of pathologic EEG activity when compared with a carefully matched group of controls with uncomplicated depression. Five of the sixteen AUDS patients in this study eventually were diagnosed as manifesting epilepsy by a consulting neurologist versus none of the sixteen patients in the depression comparison sample. No significant differences were observed between the two groups regarding pathological findings on bedside neurological examination or structural MRI scans. In the words of the authors:

We have called our study groups AUDS, pinpointing the acute and unstable depressive core symptoms. Patients displaying similar symptoms have been described in the literature with different names like "masked epilepsy," "temporal lobe syndrome," "interictal dysphoric disorder," and "subictal dysphoric disorder." These names are applied to describe conditions characterized by seizures or dysfunction presumably originating in or primarily involving mesial temporal limbic structures. Thus, a close collaboration between neurologists and psychiatrists in the evaluation and management of these patients is appropriate. However, such collaboration is rarely encountered, even in tertiary epilepsy centers, and even less in psychiatric acute wards and psychiatric intensive care units. (p. 13)

Thus, Vaaler and his colleagues described a mixed, clinical picture with many features of major depressive disorder and some features of an epileptic disorder (e.g., spells), but one that does not fit easily into any traditionally accepted diagnostic category. They also noted that 5 of 16 AUDS patients experienced brief periods with "serious affective symptoms, including intense suicidal ideations, lasting less than one hour." Other affective features included panic attacks and aggression toward others. The authors found that AUDS patients constituted 2.7% of a total of 1984 consecutive inpatient admissions (a figure that was somewhat lower than other estimates of around 10% of consecutive patients provided by Jonas [1965] for "sub-ictal neurosis" and Himmelhoch's [1984] estimate of 10% of patients with subictal dysphoric disorder among patients in an outpatient affective disorders clinic). However, this Norwegian research group did not speculate on possible etiologies for the presumed organic dysfunction of their AUDS patients.

Findings from Survey Research

Parallel to these clinical reports, survey research repeatedly has demonstrated that there is a significant association between the frequency of experiencing intermittent symptoms and previous history of head trauma in the broad normal population (Ardila et al., 1993; Roberts, Varney, Hulbert, et al., 1990; Ryan et.al., 2006). In the latter study, Ryan and colleagues administered the Iowa Interview to three groups of college-aged subjects: those with no history of TBI; those with a single episode but only alteration of consciousness; and those with brief loss of consciousness. She and her colleagues concluded:

As noted, the results . . . further support the concept of seizure phenomena as representing a continuum of neurobehavioral dysfunction. Head injury appears to be a risk factor for the endorsement of partial seizure-like phenomena. More importantly, even among mildly head injured subjects, there appears to be a continuum of symptom endorsement . . . These results need to be expanded to a clinically symptomatic head injury sample with various degrees of severity and more recent onset. (p. 290)

Studies with Children and Teens

Although we have focused thus far on adult patients, the second author has demonstrated that children and teenagers who do not fully recover from the effects of blunt-force head trauma also may display multiple episodic symptoms (e.g., Roberts, M. A., 1999; Roberts, Verduyn, Manshadi, & Hines, 1996). M. A. Roberts and colleagues reported a case study of a teenager with mild TBI that resulted in multiple episodic symptoms, cognitive deficits, and hypometabolic activity in both temporal lobes on PET scan (Roberts, Manshadi, Bushnell, & Hines, 1995). For younger children, eliciting parental report on the Pediatric Inventory of Neurobehavioral Symptoms may provide additional clinical data on the presence of episodic symptoms in addition to clinical interview of parent and child (Roberts & Furuseth, 1997).

Ancillary Features of MIND

R. J. Roberts (1999) has summarized additional history behind the currently proposed concept of MIND and described some associated clinical features of such patients. Patients who endorse multiple intermittent symptoms following head trauma frequently produce grossly abnormal profiles on the Minnesota Multiphasic Personality Inventory (MMPI, MMPI-2, or MMPI-R). Overreliance on results from personality tests such as the MMPI (and its subsequent revisions) is another reason why some clinical neuropsychologists misdiagnose the dysfunction of MIND patients as primarily psychiatric in nature or even representing malingering. The MMPI was not developed specifically for neurologic or neuropsychiatric populations (Cripe, 1999). Because they experience many troubling, intermittent symptoms, MIND patients tend to produce MMPI profiles with 6 to 10 clinically elevated scales (Roberts, Paulsen, Marchman, & Varney, 1989).

On conventional neuropsychological testing, MIND patients are likely to manifest mild-to-moderate problems with attention and memory functioning. However, roughly 65–70% of such patients fail the Dichotic Word Listening Test (Richardson, Springer, Varney, Struchen, & Roberts, 1994). Unfortunately, most neuropsychologists do not typically employ the Dichotic Word Listening Test, with the notable exception of clinicians who routinely use the Meyers Neuropsychological Battery (cf., Meyers, Roberts, Bayless, Volkert, & Evitts, 2002). This state of affairs is unfortunate for MIND patients because dichotic listening failure appears to be the most frequent, test-related deficit associated with experiencing multiple intermittent symptoms following head trauma (Roberts, R. J., 1999). Furthermore, although much research has shown that the use of anticonvulsants may be associated with cognitive dysfunction in traditional epileptic patients, open trials of treatment can ameliorate, or even normalize, dichotic listening performance in some MIND patients (Roberts, Varney, Paulsen, & Richardson, 1990).

Previous research had demonstrated that about 10–15% of MIND patients will produce clearly epileptiform EEG findings, while some 35–40% will produce a variety of EEG abnormalities (Roberts, R. J., 1999). Also, it has been demonstrated that head trauma patients who manifest an infrequent EEG pattern called "paroxysmal theta bursts" in the anterior regions of the brain are likely to endorse large numbers of intermittent symptoms on the Iowa Interview (Roberts, Franzen, & Varney, 2001; Varney, Hines, Bailey, & Roberts, 1992). If blunt-force head trauma has been involved, the individual MIND patient may or may not have deficits in the sense of smell depending upon the specifics of the blunt-force impact. However, MIND patients typically produce unremarkable results on CT and MRI scans, neurodiagnostic studies that examine gross structure of the brain—and not its function.

Interim Summary

To summarize the main points of the material presented thus far, essentially the same group of patients has been described repeatedly by various clinicians in the neuropsychiatric and brain injury literature for roughly the past five decades. However, a major barrier preventing most clinicians from identifying and treating such patients has been that different clinicians have employed a wide variety of terms to characterize such patients. Over the years, the unofficial diagnostic labels used to describe patients similar to those with MIND have included episodic dyscontrol (Monroe, 1959); subictal neurosis (Jonas, 1965); atypical psychosis (Monroe, 1982); a variant of partial seizures (Tucker et al., 1986); temporal lobe syndrome (Blumer, Heilbronn, & Himmelhoch, 1988); "atypical spells" (Tucker & Neppe, 1991); multiple partial seizure-like symptoms (Verduyn et al., 1992); a subtype of treatment-resistant depression (Varney, Garvey, Campbell, Cook, & Roberts, 1993); paroxysmal neurobehavioral disorder (Neppe & Blumer, 1998); an "epilepsy spectrum disorder" (Roberts, R. J., 1999; Taylor, 1999); subictal dysphoric disorder (Blumer, 2000); and "acute unstable depressive syndrome" (Bjork et al., 2008). Despite the plethora of different labels, the defining clinical features of such patients have remained closely consistent across the various clinical descriptions.

Evidence From the Literature on Conventional Epilepsy

At the present time, it appears that MIND is *not* generally accepted as a form of traditional epilepsy or seizure disorder by epileptologists. Epilepsy is defined as "an intermittent derangement of the nervous system due to sudden, excessive disordered discharge of cerebral neurons" (Adams & Victor, 1977). During the period of an individual seizure, the electrical activity of a pool of neurons (or even of the entire cerebrum) can fire in an inappropriately synchronous manner producing a paroxysmal (i.e., occurring in burst or as an abrupt attack) and transitory disruption of brain function. If only a restricted portion of the brain is involved, the type of epilepsy is referred to as a partial seizure disorder. Such transitory disruption of normal brain function may be rather subtle or readily apparent, even to lay observers. On the other hand, if the entire cerebrum fires in an abnormally synchronous fashion, then the type of epilepsy is referred to as a generalized seizure disorder. A generalized tonic-clonic seizure (in which the patient loses consciousness, falls to the floor, shows muscular stiffening, and then shakes rather violently) is the most obvious clinical presentation of epilepsy, one that is typically depicted in movies and television shows.

However, a number of subtypes of epilepsy exist, and not all subtypes of seizures have the same clinical features (Devinsky, 2001). On the one hand, patients with MIND generally endorse too many intermittent symptoms to be diagnosed by neurologists as manifesting a simple partial seizure disorder, a focal form of epilepsy in which a seizure patient would report one or two episodic symptoms (or auras), but not eight to twelve. On the other hand, patients with MIND generally lack the motor automatisms and periods of unconsciousness that typically characterize patients with complex partial seizure disorders, another focal form of epilepsy that often localizes to one or both temporal lobes of the brain (Roberts, Gorman, et al., 1992). Additionally, the intermittent symptoms of MIND occur unpredictably in a random-appearing fashion throughout the day, rather than occurring in the stereotyped sequences typical of complex partial seizures (e.g., an aura, then unconsciousness with motor automatisms, followed by period of post-ictal confusion). Although MIND patients often manifest brief staring spells, they lack the distinctive EEG pattern associated with *absence* or (*petit* mal) seizures, a less apparent form of generalized epilepsy than tonic-clonic seizures. However, even though MIND patients typically are not viewed as epileptic by most experts, there is major evidence from the clinical literature on patients with conventional epilepsy that is relevant to evaluating the proposition that MIND actually exists as a distinct clinical syndrome.

According to Blumer (2000), a number of epileptic patients with complex partial seizure disorders manifest an entity he has labeled "interictal dysphoric disorder." In his words:

> The histories systematically obtained from patients with chronic epilepsy at the Epi-Care Center in Memphis Tennessee, have shown that irritability, depression, three somatoform symptoms (anergia, insomnia, atypical pains), anxiety, fears, and euphoric moods are all frequently present; they are viewed as the key symptoms of interictal dysphoric disorder. (p. 10)

However, Blumer went on to observe that the same sort of complex clinical picture can also be observed in the absence of complex partial seizure disorders. When this occurs, Blumer calls this clinical entity "subictal" dysphoric disorder:

> Morel's [a prominent 19th century neuropsychiatist] early concept of "masked epilepsy". . . can be reformulated as subictal dysphoric disorder. Although the dysphoric disorder of epilepsy generally becomes manifest only some time after onset of seizures, *it may also occur in the absence of clinical seizures* [italics are ours] particularly in patients with certain brain lesions (who may or may not have an abnormal EEG).
>
> Prior to the rediscovery of the dysphoric disorder, I had described such patients as suffering from an atypical labile-pleiomorphic syndrome ("temporal lobe syndrome") requiring combined treatment with an antiepileptic and an antidepressant. These patients are not rare in my practice, but their overall frequency is difficult to assess. Himmelhoch [a neuropsychiatric collaborator with Blumer] recognized 10% of the patients in his affective disorder clinic as being in his category . . . Recognition of subictal dysphoric disorder is of particular importance, because it tends to respond very well to the combined drug treatment described above. Like interictal

dysphoric disorder, subictal dysphoric disorder requires both antiepileptics and antidepressant medications, aimed respectively at the excitatory and inhibitory components of the temporal-limbic substrate of the disturbance. Identifying the clinical syndrome of the dysphoric disorder is more productive than searching for epileptiform EEG findings, because mesial temporal seizure activity is commonly not recorded by scalp tracings. (p. 13)

Although many psychiatrists and neuropsychologists might express surprise or skepticism regarding Himmelhoch's estimate of 10% of affective disorder patients manifesting "subictal dysphoric disorder" (Blumer, Heilbronn, & Himmelhoch, 1988), Jonas (1967), who earlier coined the phrase "subictal neurosis" to characterize essentially the same group of patients, expressed a similar opinion on the proportion of his outpatient caseload that manifested this largely unrecognized clinical problem:

The subictal state is probably one of the most prevalent afflictions in modern society. Yet, so far, it has eluded the attention of physicians. Even a cursory perusal of available statistics indicates a yearly incidence of over 1,000,000 head injuries in the U.S. The injured persons will be left with . . . functionally altered neuronal cell groups capable of provoking spontaneous electrical discharges. Add to this the children who in the course of the infectious diseases either develop mild encephalitic complications or run excessively high temperatures; who fall off bicycles and receive blows to their heads in the rough and tumble plays; who were born following a traumatizing delivery; then you have an impressive reservoir of potential epileptics ranging from the entire spectrum from the mildest to the most severe cases. (p. 108)

Brewerton (1997), who reviewed much of the same literature as Blumer (2000), came to a similar conclusion regarding the occurrence of intermittent, spell-like symptoms in patients with complex partial seizures and other forms of neuropsychiatric dysfunction:

> The term "seizure" can be interpreted narrowly, in which only the most clear-cut epileptic phenomena of a psychic nature that are accompanied by observable motor or EEG components are identified as "seizure," or it can be interpreted broadly, in which a number of typical and atypical psychiatric symptoms are included as "epileptic." I argue in favor of the latter position and hope to persuade the clinical psychiatrist of the utility of a high index of suspicion. (p. 35)

Brewerton also provided 10 case histories from his own neuropsychiatric practice who responded positively to mood stabilizers with anticonvulsant properties, often in conjunction with neuroleptic medications. McAllister and his associates also reviewed the literature on complex partial seizures and depression and drew similar conclusions to those expressed by Brewerton (Greenlee, Ferrell, Kauffman, & McAllister, 2003):

> These persons may not meet criteria for MDD [Major Depressive Disorder] because of the intermittent . . . course of their illness. . . . These patients are best recognized by the paroxysmal and intermittent nature of their symptoms. (p. 411)

Thus, repeated clinical observations of individuals with conventional forms of epilepsy indicate that such epileptic patients may endorse more than one type of aura and can experience brief, aura-like experiences during the interictal periods between discrete seizures episodes. When such experiences are accompanied by clearly abnormal EEG discharges, they typically are regarded as "simple partial" seizures (i.e., sensory, motor, or affective symptoms with no change in consciousness) by traditional neurologists; however, when no apparent aura is noticed by the patients during such an electrical discharge, the abnormal brain-wave activity also may be termed a "subclinical seizure" (cf., Sperling & O'Connor, 1990).

Several groups of investigators have studied the clinical significance of multiple auras and interictal phenomena in patients with temporal lobe epilepsy. Silberman and colleagues found that patient report of a larger number of aura-type symptoms (in the absence of frank seizures) was related significantly to increased psychopathology with depression and anxiety and higher use of psychiatric treatment services (Silberman, Sussman, Skillings, & Callahan, 1994). However, similar symptoms that occurred as part of a documented seizure episode were not related to increased behavioral and emotional problems. Blume and colleagues (Manchanda, Freeland, Schaefer, McLachlan, & Blume, 2000) also studied the relationship between auras and psychiatric disorder in a sample of 144 consecutive patients with partial seizure disorder. These investigators found that epileptic patients who reported two or more auras were significantly more likely to have a psychiatric diagnosis (70.2%) when compared with epileptic patients who had only one aura (39.1%) or no auras (48.5%). Widdess-Walsh, Kotagal, Jeha, Wu, & Burgess (2007) also studied the frequency of auras in patients with partial seizure disorder. They concluded:

> Most patients who report multiple aura types have localized epilepsy in the nondominant hemisphere and are good surgical candidates. A common mechanism for multiple auras may be a spreading but restricted EEG seizure activating sequential symptomatic zones, but without ictal activation of deeper structures or contralateral spread to cause loss of awareness and amnesia for the auras. (p. 755).

Their results supported earlier work from Sperling's group (Sperling & O'Connor, 1990) also demonstrating that patients with multiple auras and subclinical seizures had a higher success rate with epilepsy surgery than did epilepsy patients without subclinical seizures and auras. A subsequent study determined that most subclinical seizures originate from the same cortical area as do full, clinical seizures; however, a minority of patients experienced subclinical seizures that emanated from different foci than did their full, clinical seizures (Zangaladze, Nei, Liporace, & Sperling, 2008).

Summary

Despite highly variable terminology, multiple neuropsychiatric clinicians have published detailed accounts of patients who report multiple, intermittent symptoms in the context of emotional lability and paroxysmal affect. Such patients frequently improved following treatment with mood stabilizers with anticonvulsant properties. We propose that the acronym MIND be employed as an abbreviation for the core features of such patients because: (a) they are *multisymptomatic*; (b) many of their symptoms are *intermittent* or episodic, as opposed to static and chronic; (c) their dysfunction in daily life appears to be brain-related and manifests in behavior, cognition, and mood (hence the term *neurobehavioral*); and (d) their symptoms are of sufficient severity that their clinical presentation constitutes a *disorder*, that is a recognizable subtype of PPCS following blunt-force head trauma.

We also believe that there is sufficient evidence to suggest that blunt-force head trauma is often a major factor contributing to the development of the symptoms of MIND. Thus, it seems likely the symptoms of MIND most often reflect an acquired disorder, rather than an inherited or genetically based syndrome. (However, vulnerability to the negative effects of head trauma may well be influenced genetically by such theoretical concepts as seizure threshold.)

Large-scale survey studies support the proposition that the report of multiple episodic symptoms is related significantly to the reported presence of a number of risk factors for cerebral dysfunction, most notably blunt-force (acceleration-deceleration) head trauma.

Studies from the clinical and research literature indicated that a MIND-like disorder (sometimes termed "interictal dysphoric disorder") occurs with considerable frequency among patients with conventional seizure disorders. However, it is not necessary for a conventional seizure disorder to be present for a neuropsychiatric patient to display a MIND-like clinical picture (termed "subictal dysphoria disorder" by Blumer [2000]).

Treatable features of MIND have been demonstrated to occur in children and teenagers following traumatic brain injury, as well as in adults.

Echoing the clinical wisdom of numerous experts, the authors suggest that the identification of patients with MIND is an important issue because such patients typically respond favorably to treatment with anticonvulsant mood stabilizers, even when there has been minimal or limited response to other types of medications.

In the next chapter, we will explore what daily life is like for adult patients who report experiencing multiple, intermittent symptoms on a daily basis.

References

Adams, R. & Victor, M. (1977). *Principles of neurology*. New York, NY: McGraw-Hill.

Ardila, A., Nino, C. R., Pulido, E., Rivera, D. B., & Vanegas, C. J. (1993). Episodic psychic symptoms in the general population. *Epilepsia, 34*, 133–140.

Bartolomei, F., Trebuchon, A., Gavaret, M., Regis, J., Wendling, F., & Chauvel, P. (2005). Acute alteration of emotional behavior in epileptic seizures is related to transient desynchrony in emotional-regulation networks. *Clinical Neurophysiology, 116*, 2472–2479.

Bjork, M. H., Sand, T., Brathen, G., Linaker, O. M., Morken, G., Nilsen, B. M., & Vaaler, A. E. (2008). Quantitative EEG findings in patients with acute, brief depression combined with other fluctuating psychiatric symptoms: A controlled study from an acute psychiatric department. *BMC Psychiatry*, *8*, 89–96.

Blumer, D. (2000). Dysphoric disorders and paroxysmal affects: Recognition and treatment of epilepsy-related psychiatric disorders. *Harvard Review of Psychiatry*, *8*, 8–17.

Blumer, D., Heilbronn, M., & Himmelhoch, J. (1988). Indications for carbamazepine in mental illness: Atypical psychiatric disorder or temporal lobe syndrome. *Comprehensive Psychiatry*, *29*, 108–122.

Brewerton, T. D. (1997). The phenomenology of psychosis associated with complex partial seizure disorder. *Annals of Clinical Psychiatry*, *9*, 31-51.

Cripe, L. I. (1999). The use of the MMPI with mild closed head injury. In N. R. Varney & R. J. Roberts (Eds.), *The evaluation and treatment of mild traumatic brain injury* (pp. 291–314). Mahwah, NJ: Lawrence Erlbaum.

Crompton, D. E., & Berkovic, S. F. (2009).The borderland of epilepsy: Clinical and molecular features of phenomena that mimic epileptic seizures. *Lancet Neurology*, *8*, 370–381.

Devinsky, O. (2001). *Epilepsy: Patient and family guide*. New York, NY: Demos Health.

Greenlee, B. A., Ferrell, R. B., Kaufman, C. I., & McAllister, T. W. (2003). Complex partial seizures and depression. *Current Psychiatry Reports*, *5*, 410–416.

Hayes, S., & Goldsmith, B. K. (1991). Psychosensory symptomatology in anticonvulsant-responsive psychiatric illness. *Annals of Clinical Psychiatry*, *3*, 108–122.

Himmelhoch, J. M. (1984). Major mood disorders related to epileptic changes. In D. Blumer, (Ed.) *Psychiatric aspects of epilepsy* (pp. 271–294). Washington, D.C.: American Psychiatric Press.

Hines, M., Swan, C., Roberts, R. J., & Varney, N. R. (1995). Characteristics and mechanisms of epilepsy spectrum disorder: An explanatory model. *Applied Neuropsychology*, *2*, 1–6.

Jonas, A. D. (1965). *Ictal and subictal neurosis*. Springfield, IL.: C. C. Thomas.

Jonas, A. D. (1967). The diagnostic and therapeutic use of diphenyl-hydantoin in the subictal state and nonepileptic dysphoria. *International Journal of Neuropsychiatry, 3*(Suppl.), 21–29.

Jonas, A. D. (1977). Ictal and subictal neurosis. *American Journal of Psychiatry, 134,* 1051–1052.

Lewis, D. O., & Pincus, J. H. (1989). Epilepsy and violence: Evidence for a neuro-psychotic-aggressive syndrome. *Journal of Neuropsychiatry and Clinical Neuroscience, 1,* 413–418.

Manchanda, R., Freeland, A., Schaefer, B., McLachlan, R. S., & Blume, W. T. (2000). Auras, seizure focus, and psychiatric disorders. *Neuropsychiatry, Neuropsychology, and Behavioral Neurology, 13,* 13–19.

Meyers, J. E., Roberts, R. J., Bayless, J. D., Volkert, K., & Evitts, P. E. (2002). Dichotic listening: Expanded norms and clinical application. *Archives of Clinical Neuropsychology, 17,* 79–90.

Monroe, R. R. (1959). Episodic behavior disorder—schizophrenia or epilepsy. *Archives of General Psychiatry, 1,* 205–214.

Monroe, R. R. (1982). Limbic ictus and atypical psychosis. *Journal of Nervous and Mental Disease, 170,* 711–716.

Neppe, V. M., & Blumer, D. (1998). *Paroxysmal neurobehavioral disorder.* Retrieved August 27, 2010, from http://www.pni.org/neuropsychiatry/seizures/PND

Persinger, M. A., & Makarec, K., (1993). Complex partial epileptic signs as a continuum from normals to epileptics: Normative data and clinical populations. *Journal of Clinical Psychology, 49,* 33–45.

Richardson, E. D., Springer, J., Varney, N. R., Struchen, M., & Roberts, R. J. (1994). Dichotic listening in the clinic: New neuropsychological applications. *Clinical Neuropsychologist, 8,* 416–429.

Roberts, M. A. (1999). Mild traumatic brain injury in children and adolescents. In N. R. Varney & R. J. Roberts (Eds.), *The evaluation and treatment of mild traumatic brain injury* (pp. 493–511). Mahwah, NJ: Lawrence Erlbaum.

Roberts, M. A., & Furuseth, A. (1997). Eliciting parental report following pediatric traumatic brain injury: Preliminary findings on the Pediatric Inventory of Neurobehavioral Symptoms. *Archives of Clinical Neuropsychology*, *12*, 449–457.

Roberts, M. A., Manshadi, F. F., Bushnell, D. L., & Hines, M. E. (1995). Neurobehavioral dysfunction following mild traumatic injury in childhood: A case report with positive findings on positron emission tomography. *Brain Injury*, *9*, 427–436.

Roberts, M. A., Verduyn, W. H., Manshadi, F. F., & Hines, M. E. (1996). Episodic symptoms in dysfunctioning children and adolescents following mild and severe traumatic brain injury. *Brain Injury, 10*, 739-747.

Roberts, R. J. (1999). Epilepsy Spectrum Disorder in the context of mild traumatic brain injury. In N. R. Varney & R. J. Roberts (Eds.), *The evaluation and treatment of mild traumatic brain injury* (pp. 409–447). Mahwah, NJ: Lawrence Erlbaum.

Roberts, R. J. (2008, December–January). Impact on the brain. *Scientific American Mind*, 50–57.

Roberts, R. J., Franzen, K., & Varney, N. R. (2001). Theta bursts, closed head injury, and partial seizure-like symptoms: A retrospective study. *Applied Neuropsychology*, *8*, 140–147.

Roberts, R. J., Gorman, L. L., Lee, G. P., Hines, M. E., Richardson, E. D., Riggle, T. A., & Varney, N. R. (1992). The phenomenology of multiple partial seizure-like symptoms without stereotyped spells: An epilepsy spectrum disorder? *Epilepsy Research*, *13*, 167–177.

Roberts, R. J., Paulsen, J. S., Marchman, J. N., & Varney, N. R. (1989). MMPI profiles of patients who endorse multiple partial seizure symptoms. *Neuropsychology*, *2*, 183–198.

Roberts, R. J., Varney, N. R., Hulbert, J. R., Paulsen, J. S., Richardson, E. D., Springer, J. A., . . . Hines, M. E. (1990). The neuropathology of everyday life: The frequency of partial seizure symptoms among normals. *Neuropsychology*, *4*, 65–86.

Roberts, R. J., Varney, N. R., Paulsen, J. S., & Richardson, E. D. (1990). Dichotic listening and complex partial seizures. *Journal of Clinical and Experimental Neuropsychology*, *12*, 448–458.

Ryan, L. M., O'Jile, J. R., Parks-Levy, J., Betz, B., Hilsabeck, R. C., & Gouvier, W. D. (2006). Complex partial seizure symptom endorsement in individuals with a history of head injury. *Archives of Clinical Neuropsychology, 21,* 287–291.

Silberman, E. K., Sussman, N. M., Skillings, G., & Callanan, M. (1994). Aura phenomenology and psychopathology: A pilot investigation. *Epilepsia, 35,* 778–784.

Sperling, M. R., & O'Connor, M. J. (1990). Auras and subclinical seizures: Characteristics and prognostic significance. *Annals of Neurology, 28,* 320–328.

Taylor, M. A. (1999). *Fundamentals of clinical neuropsychiatry.* New York, NY: Oxford University Press.

Tucker, G. J., & Neppe, V. M. (1991). Neurologic and neuropsychiatric assessment of brain injury. In H. O. Doerr & A. S. Carlin (Eds.), *Forensic neuropsychology: Legal and scientific basis* (pp. 70–85). New York, NY: Guilford Press.

Tucker, G. J., Price, T. R. P. Johnson, V. B., & McAllister, T. (1986). Phenomenology of temporal lobe dysfunction: A link to atypical psychosis—a series of cases. *Journal of Nervous and Mental Disease, 174,* 348–356.

Smoczynski, S. (1972). Clinical investigations on chronic psychic disturbances in patients with temporal lobe epilepsy. *Polish Medical Journal, 11,* 1706–1715.

Vaaler, A. E., Morken, G., Linaker, O. M., Sand, T., Kvistad, K. A., & Brathen, G. (2009). Symptoms of epilepsy and organic brain dysfunctions in patients with acute, brief depression combined with other fluctuating psychiatric symptoms: A controlled study from an acute psychiatric department. *BMC Psychiatry, 9,* 63–70.

Varney, N. R., Garvey, M., Campbell, D., Cook, B., & Roberts, R. J. (1993). Identification of treatment-resistant depressives who respond favorably to carbamazepine. *Annals of Clinical Psychiatry, 5,* 117–122.

Varney, N. R., Hines, M. E., Bailey, C., & Roberts, R. J. (1992). Neuropsychiatric correlates of theta bursts in patients with closed head injury. *Brain Injury, 6,* 449–457.

Verduyn, W. H., Hilt, J., Roberts, M. A., & Roberts, R. J. (1992). Multiple partial seizure-like symptoms following "minor" head injury. *Brain Injury, 6,* 245–260.

Widdess-Walsh, P., Kotagal, P., Jeha, L., Wu, G., & Burgess, R. (2007). Multiple auras: Clinical significance and pathophysiology. *Neurology*, *69*, 755–761.

Zangaladze, A., Nei, M., Liporace, J. D., & Sperling, M. R. (2008). Characteristics and clinical significance or subclinical seizures. *Epilepsia*, *49*, 2016–2021.

5

Living with Untreated Symptoms of MIND

The way to get people to care is to provide context.
—Chip and Dan Heath,
Made to Stick: Why Some Ideas
Survive and Others Die (2007)

Introduction

Most of us take the continuity of our thoughts and feelings more or less for granted. We assume, by and large, that we will be able to retrieve someone's name or information relevant to work when we need to do so. Barring some unforeseen occurrence, our mood later this afternoon probably will be similar to the mood we experienced earlier this morning. In short, most of us assume that our functioning in daily life will be fairly consistent and predictable (at least to ourselves) from one minute to the next. Satisfying relationships with other people, educational performance, and vocational success—all of these depend more or less on cognitive consistency, emotional stability, and the capacity to match our behaviors to the perceived demands of the social environment. Research studies have found that reduced quality of life is associated significantly with increased experiencing of mental lapses in daily life for normal individuals (Carriere, Cheyne, & Smilek, 2008) and in patients with cerebral disease (Phillips, et al., 2009).

The Distinction Between "Positive" and "Negative" Symptoms of MIND

Unfortunately, the unforeseen and disruptive occurrence of various intermittent cognitive, sensory, and emotional symptoms makes coping with daily life considerably less predictable for patients with MIND following mild TBI. One key to understanding the impact of MIND on daily functioning is to remember that it is associated with multiple *interruptions* and *lapses* in normal brain function. For a few seconds or even a few minutes, a patient with MIND may experience the olfactory illusion of an unpleasant odor (e.g., kitty litter, electrical fire) for which there is no cause and that no one around them smells. When such a transitory sensory illusion intrudes into consciousness, the patient experiencing the illusion likely is to be at least momentarily distracted from his or her previous focus of attention. Similarly, when specifically asked, a patient with mild blunt-force TBI may admit to experiencing visual illusions of movement or a shadowy-like figure, like a mouse or a large cockroach, on one side of peripheral vision, but then the patient turns his head to the side only to find that nothing is there. Such false perceptions, when they occur in the context of conventional epilepsy, are called "psycho-sensory" illusions or "unformed hallucinations" to distinguish them from the more complex and persistent hallucinatory symptoms associated with primary psychiatric disorders, such as schizophrenia.

False sensory illusions are categorized as *positive symptoms*, not because they are positive or pleasing to experience, but because a person's consciousness registers a positive phenomenon, such as a particular foul taste or ringing in the ears, that does not reflect the effects of an actual physical stimulus upon the sense organs. One reason why some MIND patients may be disinclined to describe the full range of sensory illusions they experience is the popular belief that all sensory illusions and hallucinations necessarily are associated with primary psychotic disorders, such as schizophrenia and mania. This is particularly true for teens and young adults who experience symptoms of MIND. Fairly or unfairly, one stereotype of individuals with severe psychiatric disorders is that the sufferers hear things or see things that are not really there. One effect of this common misattribution ("I must be going crazy!") is that some TBI patients are reluctant to spontaneously describe their multiple sensory illusions or unformed hallucinations to family members or care providers. When interviewing such reluctant patients, bland reassurance that they are not going crazy (but that certain symptoms may make them *feel* as if they are going crazy) may prove helpful for encouraging them to report on the full range of symptoms that they are actually experiencing.

Other symptoms exhibited by MIND patients, such as cognitive lapses and memory gaps, are predominantly *negative symptoms*, in that their minds cease to function normally for brief periods of time or partially cut-out on them. Rather than full-fledged black-outs (e.g., loss of consciousness) that would be associated with a clear seizure disorder, such symptoms are more like electrical brown-outs that occur when everyone comes home at the same time on an extremely hot day and begins to use their air conditioners or other electrical appliances. The electric lights or the picture on the TV may dim or sputter, but the power does not go off completely. Occasionally patients or families actually have selected a colloquial name for describing such negative symptoms, such as "short-circuits," "spacing off," "brain-farts," or "walk-abouts."

Word-finding and name-retrieval lapses can be awkward in social settings such as work and school, with the individual left stammering, asking for help, or trying to gloss over a lapse. (One Army officer who tended to have embarrassing, name-retrieval lapses in front of his soldiers described the phenomena as "coming up blank" and then having to "flip through my mental

Rolodex" to try to retrieve the correct name.) Similarly, MIND patients may space off or fail to recall part or all of a previous conversation in which they participated; they may even argue with a family member or co-worker that the conversation never actually took place ("You never told me that!"). Patients may go blank or switch topics in the middle of an ongoing conversation with no warning or transition. One spouse, borrowing on terminology from bidding the card game Bridge, described her husband's sudden changes in the topic of conversation as "jump-shifts." Some MIND patients may need to pull to the side of the road and stop driving briefly because a familiar route they are on somehow no longer looks like it should (i.e., *jamais vu*— the opposite of *déjà vu*). Such lapses in daily functioning can become so annoying that patients older than 50 can worry about the possible onset of early Alzheimer's disease, whereas younger patients sometimes inquire about the possible development of a "late-onset" attention deficit disorder.

Affective (Emotional) Symptoms of MIND

In addition to unpredictable sensory illusions and mental lapses, MIND patients also frequently report experiencing abrupt, ego-dystonic mood-swings consisting of sadness, anger outbursts, or spells of untriggered panic and anxiety—abrupt mood swings that seem to come and go for no apparent reason. A patient may yell vociferously at a family member for basically no reason and then forget that the episode occurred half an hour later. For example, one brain-injured Vietnam combat veteran became enraged at his truck for no apparent reason, started beating it with a large hammer, and then walked past his stunned family members and went indoors to take a nap. If there is an eliciting stimulus for a rage outburst, the patient's emotional reaction may be way out of proportion to the event that provoked the outburst (e.g., getting upset and screaming for five minutes because a child spilled a glass of milk on the floor). Although circumstances vary, it is usually episodes of intense anger that are most troubling to the family members of patients with MIND. Often, such patients express genuine remorse following the episode. They may apologize or act stunned when confronted with the full impact of their rage outbursts by others. If a history of past head trauma has gone unrecognized by care providers, some individuals with MIND may receive the psychiatric diagnosis of Intermittent Explosive Disorder.

In addition to anger outbursts, blunt-force, mild TBI patients with MIND may complain of feeling abruptly more depressed, unhappy, or even suicidal in the absence of any clear reason or obvious, eliciting life event. Such mood changes can be profound and puzzling because of the lack of a coherent explanation as to why the person should feel that way. Often, the abnormal sad or depressed mood goes away as mysteriously as it began— for no apparent reason. Patients who develop symptoms of MIND following blunt-force head trauma often meet criteria for a major depressive episode, and, if the care provider is not aware of a history of head trauma, may receive a diagnosis of primary depression. On the other hand, if the care provider is aware of a history of head trauma and believes that a given patient's depressed mood is secondary to head trauma, then the diagnosis of mood disorder secondary to a general medical condition also may be used. Because MIND patients tend to have limited positive response to SSRI antidepressant medications, some psychiatrists tend to regard them as manifesting a form of treatment-resistant depression. Finally, some MIND patients also may manifest a persistent, low-level, chronic dysphoria in addition to their brief untriggered bouts of depressed mood—a form of "double depression" (Keller & Shapiro, 1982).

In addition to spell-like problems with rage and depressed mood, discrete episodes of panic or extreme anxiety may overwhelm an individual with MIND for no apparent reason. These episodes do not appear to be triggered by any particular fear-provoking stimuli and tend to emerge out of the blue, and treatment for traditional panic attacks with antidepressant medications typically produces little or no relief. When interviewing combat veterans and other traumatized patients, care needs to be taken to differentiate *untriggered*, ego-dystonic spells of anxiety from arousal associated with the re-experiencing of traumatic events that has been elicited or triggered by a specific stimulus (e.g., thunder or fireworks sounding similar to artillery fire).

Relatives and friends typically describe individuals with MIND as excessively moody or more emotionally labile than they were prior to sustaining blunt-force head trauma. As mentioned previously, when patients are faced with unexplained affective instability, in addition to intermittent psycho-sensory and cognitive symptoms, a number of MIND patients can be reluctant to express the full range of their concerns to their health-care providers—lest the providers think them "crazy." Many military or law enforcement personnel, who have been trained to adapt and overcome all obstacles, try to minimize, ignore, or deny their symptoms as a means of coping with them. Sometimes patients (or family members) may report the presence of symptoms fairly convincingly but misattribute them to other causes (e.g., PTSD, a stressful divorce, exposure to toxins like Agent Orange, or the stress of schoolwork in a child with unrecognized learning disabilities).

Factors That Can Complicate the Diagnostic Process

When MIND patients repeatedly have failed to benefit from (or have derived limited benefit from) treatment with conventional psychotropic medications or cognitive-behavior therapy, both care providers and patients can become understandably discouraged. In many cases, the onset or recognition of significant symptoms may not *immediately* follow the occurrence of head trauma but may be delayed by weeks or months, thereby obscuring the causative relationship between the acute head trauma and the development of episodic symptoms of MIND.

If the prefrontal region of the brain, which is thought to be involved in mediating so-called executive functions, also has been damaged by blunt-force trauma, a mild TBI patient may have difficulty providing a coherent medical history to even the most well-intentioned care provider. In the words of one neurologist, "If there's something wrong with the history, and the history taker is competent, then there's most likely something wrong with the patient." Patients with prefrontal damage or dysfunction also may admit to the presence of symptoms ("Yeah, that happens") but have difficulty providing clear frequency estimates on the Iowa Interview ("Oh, not that often . . . "). Or they may fail to comprehend the content or mishear a direct question, provide an answer based upon what they thought the question was about, and then later appear to be contradicting themselves.

It was for these reasons that the decision was made to present the content of the Iowa Interview as a semi-structured *interview* rather than a self-administered questionnaire. We discourage clinicians from using the items on the Iowa Interview as a self-rating scale for patients because a good degree of professional judgment based upon clinical experience with actual patients generally is required to separate intermittent symptoms from similar symptoms due to other causes. For example, haptic (tactile) illusions are qualitatively different from the effects of chronic neuropathies, but both can produce tingling in the extremities. However, the sensations produced by peripheral neuropathies are more or less constant rather than intermittent. Similarly, Vietnam combat veterans may describe having "olfactory flashbacks" when, in fact, they are experiencing untriggered olfactory illusions. Follow-up questions and sound clinical judgment are required to make these subtle distinctions.

When their brains work properly, the minds of blunt-force TBI patients with MIND function reasonably well; however, when their brains misfire, the mental, emotional, and behavioral functioning of a MIND patient becomes temporarily unreliable —seemingly for no apparent reason. An adult may walk to the garage or toolshed to get a certain tool and forget what he had gone after by the time he arrives at his destination. A teenager may get sent to the local grocery store to pick up three items for his parent, drive to the store, and then have to use his cell phone to have the same instructions repeated. Despite adequate word-identification skills, the grades of a high-school student with MIND may plummet because the student forgets the content of reading a textbook by the time she gets to the bottom of the page. Adults who have been avid recreational readers all their lives may actually quit reading altogether due to the frustration of frequently forgetting the content of what has just been read.

An Analogy Between the Disrupted MIND and an Unreliable Computer

In this high-tech age, analogies often are drawn between the human mind and a computer. Just imagine what it would be like to have purchased a new home computer, but one that ran correctly only 97% of the time. The other 3% of the time the computer malfunctioned in various unpredictable ways. For a few seconds at a time, the mouse may go dead without any warning. Sometimes the modem links up to the correct Internet site, but occasionally it doesn't. Major parts of a word-processed manuscript get saved, but other small portions are trashed or deleted. Occasionally, the computer's speakers produce static for a few minutes, or the computer screen grows dim or fuzzy. Under such circumstances, very little meaningful work could be accomplished —even though the computer ran correctly the vast majority of the time. To the extent that this computer analogy is valid, it is not surprising that many MIND patients (like Jane in Chapter 2), continue to complain of active problems and push for effective treatment of their intermittent symptoms.

Now add to this scenario the unpredictable spells of irritability, depressed mood, and/or extreme anxiety that MIND patients may experience. Unlike most of us, patients with such extreme mood swings cannot necessarily predict what sort of mood they will be in two hours into the future. Such variability of mood can produce adjustment issues in the best of families. In particular, alternating cycles of rage outbursts followed by social withdrawal due to depression, anxiety, or guilt are difficult for families to cope with and to understand.

Jonas (1965) eloquently described the plight of his patients with subictal neurosis (his term for what the present authors call MIND):

> The abnormal manifestations can so interpose themselves that a patient no longer thinks of himself as a functioning entity, but more nearly as a self on the verge of disintegration. Since the [sub-] ictal activity is paroxysmal and short-lasting, it becomes unreal in retrospect. The initial detachment alternates with a fear of insanity, and thus it becomes almost a necessity for the individual to lead a well-circumscribed life in which nothing is left to chance. Over a period of a few years, the self-imposed restrictions, the rigid rules, all lead to a functional paralysis. The individual can no longer participate in the social goals of his environment. His growing sense of inadequacy and embarrassment further intensifies the process of alienation. The anticipation of feeling himself passing from a real world into a hazy, twilight state in which his actions and mental processes have become distorted leads to severe anxiety. He faces a condition which he can neither describe, define nor understand. (p. 25)

Although written more than four decades ago, the words of Jonas (1965) remain relevant today. Complicating the clinical situation of the patient with MIND, many such individuals are reticent to describe their full range of symptoms for fear of feeling embarrassed, crazy, or dismissed by their care providers.

> On his way to the physician, the worried individual will ponder what to say, with thoughts along these lines: "Well, I just can't tell him I had a funny feeling inside my head that hit me suddenly the other day, for no good reason. I had also a little nausea and some pressure in the stomach. I feel a little dizzy, but it wasn't like falling

down, more like something turning in my head. But I can just see the doctor giving me that puzzled look, wondering why I'm troubling him with such trivialities. He'll probably tell me I shouldn't work so hard." (p. 17)

Jonas continued:

I was consistently struck by the obvious reluctance of these patients to discuss the . . . subictal states. Hesitation in speech, a gesture of dismissal, or an exasperated "I don't know what to tell you," "I don't know how to say it," or "It's the damnedest thing and I only wish I could describe it," were commonplace. Repeated encouragement to convey the essence of the sensations they felt, the emotional impact of the bizarre and inchoate reverberations, eventually enabled most of these individuals to communicate the nature of their most intimate perceptions. (p. 20)

Advantages of a Structured Interview

One obvious advantage of using a semi-structured interview to assess intermittent symptoms is that the structure tends to normalize the evaluation process for the patient simply because the interviewer is inquiring about episodic phenomena in a matter-of-fact way.

It is important to understand at this point that MIND patients virtually never endorse experiencing all of the 40 symptoms on the Iowa Interview. Nor do all MIND patients experience the exact same symptoms with similar frequencies. For example, some MIND patients may not suffer from rage outbursts with a clinically significant frequency. Other MIND patients may not experience episodes when they briefly garble their speech or mangle their words. Still others may lack the illusion of perceiving a foul taste in their mouths for a few minutes at a time for no apparent reason. Just as no two instances of head injury are identical, the responses of head-trauma patients to the items on the Iowa Interview also are highly individualized. Thus, the evaluating clinician is encouraged to administer and score the entire Iowa Interview and compare the patient's total frequency of all symptoms on the interview with normative standards, rather than basing clinical decisions on the presence or absence of just one or two intermittent symptoms.

In the next chapter, we discuss various pharmacological treatment issues for patients who develop symptoms of MIND following blunt-force head trauma.

References

Carriere, J. S., Cheyne, J. A., & Smilek, D. (2008). Everyday attention and memory failures: The affective consequences of mindlessness. *Consciousness and Cognition, 17,* 835–847.

Heath, C., & Heath, D. (2007). *Made to stick: Why some ideas survive and others die.* New York, NY: Random House.

Jonas, A. D. (1965). *Ictal and subictal neurosis.* Springfield, IL: Charles C. Thomas.

Keller, M. B., & Shapiro, R. W. (1982). "Double depression": Superimposition of acute depressive episodes on chronic depressive disorders. *American Journal of Psychiatry, 139,* 438–442.

Phillips, L. H., Saldias, A., McCarrey, A., Henry, J. D., Scott, C., Summers, F., & Whyte, M. (2009). Attentional lapses, emotional regulation, and quality of life in multiple sclerosis. *British Journal of Clinical Psychology, 48,* 101–106.

6

Reviewing the Evidence of Treatment Efficacy

Without therapeutic enthusiasm, there would be no innovation, and without skepticism, there would be no proof.

—Vladimir Hachinski (Quoted in Fogel, Duffy, McNamara, & Salloway, 1992, p. 458)

The joy of good clinical work is the ability to participate in a client's personal healing. But along with the potential for great impact comes a tremendous responsibility. . . . The first rule is "Do no harm," yet we harm when we do not prepare enough to do our best. Our clients place their lives and their psyches . . . in our care. Only our highest integrity, our most educated level of skill, and our profound compassion should answer their need.

—Francine Shapiro (2001, p. 382)

Introduction

This chapter begins with a disclaimer. The first two authors of this book are both Ph.D.-level clinical neuropsychologists—and *not* physicians. Therefore, the two primary authors are not permitted legally to prescribe any sort of medication in our clinical practices. The content of this chapter comes largely from three sources: (1) the available research literature concerning pharmacological treatment of mild TBI patients; (2) our clinical experiences observing how many different physicians practice when assessing and treating patients with MIND; and (3) the neuropsychiatric expertise of our collaborator, William Sheehan, M.D., a board-certified and licensed psychiatrist.

The prescription of any medication is a *medical* decision and *not* a neuropsychological decision; however, the diagnostic impressions, test findings, and systematic behavioral observations of ancillary health-care professionals, such as neuropsychologists, can assist physicians in the process of selecting of a particular approach for treating the individual patient.

Recommendations of Expert Clinicians

In Chapter 4, we established that two prominent neuropsychiatrists, Gary Tucker and Michael Alan Taylor, have recommended that patients with multiple intermittent symptoms be given trials on mood-stabilizing medications with anticonvulsant properties. Tucker and colleagues (Tucker, Price, Johnson, & McAllister, 1986) initially theorized that these patients manifested a variant of epilepsy, but in his later writings, Tucker appeared to pull back from this notion somewhat (Tucker, 1998). Nevertheless, he continued to recommend strategic trials of such medications for MIND-like patients. Taylor (1999) also observed that such patients tend to benefit from pharmacological treatment with medications similar to those used to treat seizures, whether or not they actually suffered from a type of seizure disorder.

Two of the most important clinical questions in the practice of the healing arts are as follows:

1. "What is the nature of the dysfunction exhibited by the patient?"
2. "What can be done to help the patient?"(cf., Stapert, 2009).

Perhaps the clearest and most forceful opinion regarding pharmacological treatment of poly-symptomatic patients following head injury comes from another prominent neuropsychiatrist, Barry S. Fogel (Tierney & Fogel, 1995). Dr. Fogel is a self-described therapeutic "enthusiast" (Fogel, Duffy, McNamara, & Salloway, 1992) who suggests that much time and money can be spent trying to determine whether or not a patient with multiple intermittent symptoms following head injury is "epileptic" or not. Fogel has argued that attempting a strategic trial of treatment to determine whether a patient with multiple intermittent symptoms improves on a mood stabilizer with anticonvulsant properties is more likely to pay clinical dividends than conducting an expensive and elusive search for a clearly epileptic form of EEG abnormality.

Working independently of both Tucker and Taylor, Tierney and Fogel wrote in 1995:

> The mood-stabilizing antiepileptic drugs carbamazepine and valproic acid should be considered as treatment for mood instability, impulsivity, and episodic neurologic symptoms, particularly those that have a sudden onset. Their efficacy as symptomatic therapies in patients with TBI has much anecdotal support but essentially no confirmation by placebo-controlled studies. However, it is clear that they can help patients whose symptoms do not warrant a diagnosis of epilepsy as well as people with normal or abnormal, but non-epileptiform, electroencephalograms. . . . In many cases, much time and money are spent in pursuit of an EEG abnormality, when the more important question of whether antiepileptic drugs would help would be better answered by a planned clinical trial with systematic assessment of target symptoms. (p. 307)

Interestingly, Blumer (2000), a prominent American epileptologist, also has emphasized that making the correct clinical diagnosis is often more important than chasing after elusive EEG abnormalities.

> Recognition of subictal dysphoric disorder is of particular importance, because it tends to respond very well to the

> combined drug therapy described above [i.e., the combi-
> nation of an anticonvulsant mood-stabilizer and an anti-
> depressant]. . . . Identifying the clinical syndrome of the
> [subictal] dysphoric disorder is more productive than
> searching for epileptiform EEG findings, because mesial
> temporal seizure activity is not commonly recorded by
> scalp [EEG] tracings. (p. 13)

Although this would appear to be straightforward guidance,
many physicians we have observed choose not to follow such
guidance for a variety of reasons.

As Fogel himself has acknowledged, significant differences
exist among care providers in the degree to which they are will-
ing to prescribe in cases that are not clear cut. Those who are
on the more conservative end of the spectrum Fogel described
as therapeutic "skeptics;" those on the more liberal end, Fogel
termed therapeutic "enthusiasts." Without liberal enthusiasts,
Fogel noted, there would be little or no innovation; without conservative skeptics to ensure that research is conducted properly
and evaluated, there would be less stringent verification. Within
a diverse clinical area, such as the treatment of brain injury,
Fogel and his colleagues observed that there should be room for
both therapeutic activism and skepticism (Fogel et al., 1992),
especially in understudied areas such as the pharmacological
treatment of PPCS and persistent mild TBI.

In the 1995 quotation from Tierney and Fogel provided previously, they acknowledged that there had been no placebo-
controlled trials of medication for treating the longer term effects
of mild TBI. Unfortunately, this statement is almost as true today
as it was back in 1995. Recently, neuropsychiatrists have reviewed
the existing literature, which does provide some fairly solid evidence for the use of a certain class of antidepressant medication,
SSRIs (Selective Serotonin Re-uptake Inhibitors), for treating post-
TBI depression (Fann, Hart, & Schomer, 2009; Silver, McAllister,
& Arciniegas, 2009). For instance, Ashman et al. (2009), conducted
a recent randomized controlled trial of Sertraline (Zoloft), which
demonstrated that this SSRI antidepressant was effective in treating

depressed mood following mild traumatic brain injury. However, no similar double-blind, placebo-controlled study exists for using either mood stabilizer, carbamazepine or valproic acid, for treating the symptoms of MIND following blunt-force head trauma.

In a double-blind, placebo-controlled study, an inert substance (the placebo) is compared against an active medication, and both the patients and prescribing physicians are blind to which patients are receiving the placebo and which are receiving the active drug. Patients are assigned at random to either the treatment group or the control group (which typically receives a placebo); thus, this also is what is meant by the phrase "randomized controlled trial." At the end of such a study, the code is broken, and the data from both groups are analyzed statistically to determine whether the active drug was more effective than the placebo in treating the condition (e.g., depression following traumatic brain injury) that is being targeted.

Generally speaking, it requires at least one convincing double-blind, placebo-controlled study before some clinicians feel comfortable prescribing a medication for a particular condition or syndrome. The major, demonstrated use(s) of given medications are referred to as "approved" by the Food and Drug Administration. If a physician were to prescribe a medication (approved for treating epileptic seizures) for treating the mood swings and intermittent symptoms of MIND following head injury, that physician would be engaging in an "off-label" application (or nonapproved use) of the particular medication, based upon his judgment and knowledge of the clinical literature. Both carbamazepine (Tegretol) and valproic acid (Depakote, Divalproex) have been approved primarily as anticonvulsant drugs used to treat epilepsy. They also have been used widely by psychiatrists to treat bipolar affective disorder. Furthermore, because both medications can produce fairly rare, but medically serious, side effects, more conservative physicians are understandably concerned about using either medication for an off-label application with TBI patients.

Nevertheless, other forms of evidence in addition to double-blind, placebo-controlled trials of a medication are available, such as (a) published guidelines from expert clinicians; (b) the results from open-trials of medication (a case series); and (c) intensive case studies, which supports Tierney and Fogel's (1995) assertion that mood stabilizers with anticonvulsant properties frequently are helpful for treating the MIND-like symptoms of head trauma patients with brain injuries. We will review these three types of supporting information in the following sections.

Clinical Recommendations and Guidelines

Zappala and Cameron (1990) have recommended that clinicians consider the use of carbamazepine for treating "subictal and interictal temporal lobe phenomena" following traumatic brain injury:

> Because these symptoms are often amenable to treatment, sometimes with dramatic results, clinicians should keep a high index of suspicion for temporal lobe dysfunction in traumatic brain injury. . . . Carbamazepine has been demonstrated to be effective not only for generalized seizures or for typical temporal lobe seizures, but also for a range of psychiatric-like disorders commonly seen after . . . head trauma, even in the presence of a normal EEG. . . . Failure to recognize these symptoms as a potentially treatable neurologic condition may reduce their potential for participating in a rehabilitation program and for a good outcome. Treatment with carbamazepine can frequently help to eradicate or moderate these symptoms, while helping the patient to realize his or her maximum potential in a multidisciplinary rehabilitation program. (p. 5)

Blumer, Montouris, and Davies (2004) expressed similar support for pharmacological treatment of dysphoria, rage, and intermittent symptoms of the MIND-like condition they called "subictal dysphoric disorder."

> Psychiatrists . . . must become able to recognize, among their own patients, the presence of a subictal dysphoric disorder that requires . . . combined treatment with antidepressant and antiepileptic medications. (p. 826)

In calling attention to the factors that predict good response to carabamazepine, Blumer, Heilbronn, and Himmelhoch (1988) asserted, "A wide range of atypical, labile-pleiomorphic psychiatric disorders respond specifically to carbmazepine" (p. 108). Varney and colleagues (1993) reached a similar conclusion: " . . . our preliminary observations suggest that a salient patient variable, namely, the reported presence of multiple seizure-like symptoms, may ultimately prove useful in identifying a subgroup of potentially refractory patients for whom carbamazepine therapy should be considered" (p. 120).

Neppe and Tucker (1994) likewise emphasized the use of anticonvulsant mood-stabilizers for patients with multiple, spell-like symptoms:

> In psychiatry particularly, patients at times have episodes that are extremely difficult to interpret. The episodes may be very short-lived, lasting second or minutes, but on occasion can last for days. Such patients behave out of character and usually exhibit a lability of affect that is profound, with disturbances ranging from depression through mania. . . . We have called such episodes *spells* to obviate debate as to whether they are truly ictal.
>
> In such episodes, EEGs may not reveal any additional information, or these patients may have temporal lobe spikes or at least slowing in the temporal lobe. Such episodes have been labeled *temporal lobe epilepsy* or *atypical complex partial seizures*. The neurologists justifiably have debated whether these are "real" seizures. The patients may respond to anticonvulsant medication, and trials of anticonvulsants are needed. In our experience, many of these patients respond well to carbamazepine (Tegretol particularly), phenytoin (Dilantin), or valproate

(Depakene, Depakote). It is possible that these patients occasionally may respond to a short course of anticonvulsant therapy and not require permanent treatment. . . . This is a major transition area between psychiatry and neurology. (pp. 415–416)

One year following Neppe and Tucker's article, Hines and colleagues (Hines, Swan, Roberts, & Varney, 1995) also reviewed the literature on patients with "epilepsy spectrum disorder" in the process of developing an explanatory, physiological model of MIND-like symptoms:

Unlike patients with classic complex partial seizure disorders, ESD ("epilepsy spectrum disorder," [or MIND] patients do not experience their symptoms in a predictable stereotypic sequence. The patient with ESD is likely to experience each symptom in a seemingly random fashion, one or two at a time. In the majority of cases, the standard EEGs obtained from ESD patients are typically interpreted as being within normal limits or as showing abnormalities not clearly epileptiform in nature. Nevertheless, a clear majority respond well to anticonvulsant medications, particularly carbamazepine and valproic acid, even when there has been a history of profound treatment failure with more traditional psychotropic medications . . . (p. 1)

More recently, Lux (2007) has recommended the use of anticonvulsant mood stabilizers for treating sudden anger and impulsive aggression following brain injury, based upon his review of the brain trauma literature and his clinical experiences at treating military personnel at Walter Reed Army Medical Center.

One important additional chronic behavioral condition that can develop after TBI, particularly in persons with known temporal lobe lesions, is the syndrome of episodic dyscontrol or intermittent explosive disorder. Patients with this syndrome are prone to rage attacks, i.e., brief outbursts of extreme anger, associated with agitated, aggressive, and/or violent behavior. The outbursts have a paroxysmal quality and may occur with little or no provocation. . . . The condition has been reported to respond to the psychotropic anticonvulsants carbamazepine and valproic acid. (p. 956)

Similarly, Anderson (2008) has suggested that clinicians consider the use of valproic acid and carbamazepine to treat affective instability and impulsive aggression following blast-exposure. Additionally, the joint Veterans Affairs/Department of Defense clinical practice guidelines on the "Management of Concussion/ mild Traumatic Brain Injury" suggest consideration of antiepileptic medications *and* SSRI antidepressants for the management of depressed mood with "irritability" and "poor frustration tolerance" (Department of Defense, 2009, p. 44).

Recently, the actual practices of physiatrists (physicians who specialize in rehabilitation medicine) were surveyed by Francisco and his associates (Francisco, Walker, Zasler, & Bouffard, 2007). Among the most common prescription medications chosen by specialists included the use of valproic acid and carbamazepine for controlling agitation; the use of valproic acid for treating anger; the use of valproic acid for treating chronic irritability; and the use of both valproic acid and carbamazepine for treating emotional lability following brain injury. In contrast, SSRI antidepressants were the most common choices to treat uncomplicated depression following brain injury. In a chart-review study, Han and her associates found that anticonvulsants were the second most common class of medications prescribed to TBI patients (27%), following only antianxiety and antidepressants (43%) (Han, Craig, Rutner, Kapoor, Ciufferda, & Suchoff 2008). They noted:

Medications in the antihypertensive, antidepressant, and anticonvulsant categories may be prescribed to patients with TBI . . . for the off-label treatment of the following conditions: attention, arousal, aggression, agitation, restlessness, cognition, and vestibular disorders. (p. 257)

Thus, in real-world contexts, it seems apparent that many physicians use anticonvulsant mood stabilizers for off-label applications when caring for patients with traumatic brain injury.

Ratcliff and colleagues (Yasseen, Colantonio, & Ratcliff, 2008) interviewed 306 patients with moderate-to-severe TBI who had been treated and discharged from a large rehabilitation unit over a 16-year period. The patients and their families provided information on their current use of prescription medications. The most frequently prescribed class of medication was anticonvulsants (25.9 %), followed by antidepressants (8.2%), painkillers (8.2%), and antianxiety medications (5.9%). The authors noted:

Anti-convulsant medications are used for multiple purposes and indications; however, this study was limited in determining these indications . . . administration of anticonvulsants is routine for persons with recent incidents of TBI for the control of seizures, pain, mood stabilization and aggression . . . the prolonged use of prescription anticonvulsants in persons with TBI could be due to a variety of factors which include seizure control and neuropathic pain. All of these factors could possibly be a result of [a] TBI incident. (p. 756)

Thus, data from three separate studies indicate that anticonvulsant medications clearly are among the types of drugs prescribed to persons with TBI in the post-acute or maintenance stages of recovery.

Case Series

Jonas (1967b) reported on the clinical utility of the anticonvulsant phenytoin (Dilantin) for treating the multiple, intermittent symptoms and dysphoric moods of 112 patients with subictal neurosis. The EEG findings from these patients were either normal or not clearly characteristic of a conventional epileptic disorder. These patients were treated with open nonblind trials of phenytoin. Of 112 such patients treated, 59% showed at least moderate symptom-relief from treatment, and 18% manifested markedly improved functioning. As one postgraduate student with excellent treatment response reported:

> I now understand the difficulty I had with my mind. Ordinarily, I would hear the sound of the words, but there was a gap between the sound and the meaning. It was as if the words had to travel a given distance before I could understand it. After taking one capsule, this distance vanishes. (p. S26)

In addition to a reduction in symptoms and improvement in mood, Jonas's patients with good response reportedly become more amenable to psychological interventions such as psychotherapy. Jonas considered the possibility that his results could be due to a placebo effect, but ended up discounting this logical possibility as unlikely, in part because subictal patients treated with psychotropic medications other than phenytoin did not manifest similar levels of reported clinical improvement. (More recently approved anticonvulsants, such as carbamazepine and valproic acid, were not available to Jonas because they had not yet been approved for use at the time he started studying his case series.)

Probably the best-known case series of treated MIND-like patients remains that of Tucker, Price, Johnson, and McAllister (1986). Of a total of 20 treatment-refractory patients, 18 manifested a favorable treatment response with anticonvulsant medication. Eight of the twenty patients had "complete clearing" of their symptoms. In this case series, the medications used to treat various patients were phenytoin, carbamazepine, and valproic acid (i.e., Dilantin, Tegretol, and Depakote, respectively). That three different anticonvulsant medications could produce favorable outcomes in individual patients suggested that it was likely to be the *anti-epileptic* properties of these three medications, which were responsible for symptom-reduction and improved mood. It should be noted that all patients in this case series had a history of at least one abnormal (but not clearly epileptiform) EEG.

Working independently of Tucker's group, Roberts and his associates discovered that defective dichotic listening performance was a frequent finding in patients with multiple partial seizure-like symptoms (Roberts, Varney, Paulsen, & Richardson, 1990). Eighteen of the twenty-four patients in this case series were re-evaluated following open trials of treatment with carbamazepine. The average number of intermittent symptoms in this treated subgroup was significantly lower than it had been at baseline. For the 12 patients who completed MMPI protocols before and after treatment, there was a significant decrease in the number of clinically significant scale elevations. Considering all treated patients, all mean dichotic listening indices were significantly higher (i.e., better cognitive performance) following treatment with carbamazepine. The authors concluded: " . . . It was observed that even grossly impaired dichotic listening performance could be normalized or substantially improved when seizure symptoms were successfully treated . . . " (p. 457).

In a separate case series of 13 patients with treatment-refractory depression and a clinically significant number of episodic symptoms, Roberts's group found that 11 of the 13 patients demonstrated significant improvement on the Beck and Hamilton depression rating scales (Varney, Garvey, Cook, Campbell, & Roberts, 1993). Six patients were judged to manifest substantial improvement by the rating psychiatrist, five showed moderate improvements, and the remaining two patients were only minimally improved. Thus, 85% percent of this case series displayed at least moderate improvement following treatment with carbamazepine.

As discussed earlier, Verduyn, Hilt, Roberts, and Roberts (1992) described a series of 17 patients who developed multiple, partial seizure-like symptoms after sustaining minor closed head trauma. All but two patients in this case series were given open trials of carbamazepine or valproic acid. Twelve of the fifteen treated patients (80%) were judged to have exhibited at least moderate improvement on an anticonvulsant mood stabilizer. However, the authors noted that reduction in the frequency of episodic symptoms was not always associated with return to full functional status in everyday life; this was largely because a number of the patients in this case series also manifested significant deficits in executive function as well as some residual intermittent symptoms.

Wroblewski, Joseph, Kupfer, and Kalliel (1997) published a series of five cases in which open trials of valproic acid were used to target dysphoric mood and aggressive behavior.

> In all cases valproic acid was effective after other pharmacological interventions were not. Also, the addition of valproic acid was followed by neurobehavioral improvement rather quickly, often within 1–2 weeks. Advantages of valproic acid, in addition to its possible unique efficacy, include a lower propensity towards sedation and cognitive impairment, and thus a more robust potential for rehabilitation participation. Behaviours associated with affective disorder ranging along the affective spectrum from depression to dysphoric mania may be particularly amenable to valproic acid. The drug may also be beneficial in some cases in which another psychotropic anticonvulsant, carbamazepine, was not. (p. 37)

Persinger (2000) reported on a case series of 14 patients who had sustained brain traumas during motor vehicle accidents and reported abnormally high scores on an early version of the Iowa Interview. Of these 14 treated cases treated with carbamazepine, 12 (86%) reported that " . . . within a few weeks after treatment they experienced marked reductions in the incidence of sudden confusion and depression, increased attention and focus, and either elimination or attenuation of an aversive sensed presence" (p. 37). Persinger argued that " . . . many of the debilitating symptoms that persist for months to years after a traumatic brain injury may be neuro-electric in nature rather than 'psychological responses' to having been injured" (p. 37).

Kim and Humaran (2002) performed a retrospective chart review on 11 patients with a remote history of acquired brain injury. These patients were highly heterogeneous and manifested a wide variety of psychiatric symptoms. All patients were judged to be significantly improved, and none experienced adverse side effects. The authors concluded:

> Divalproex sodium, either alone or in combination with other psychotropic medications, appears to be well-tolerated and effective in reducing a broad range of neurobehavioral symptoms in community-dwelling patients with ABI [acquired brain injury]. We suggest that the anti-kindling effects rather than a specific anti-manic effect of Divalproex is responsible for its broad range of benefits, and that limbic kindling may be responsible for a wide variety of ABI-induced psychopathology. (p. 105)

The word "anti-kindling" in the preceding quotation refers to the potential for preventing (or arresting) the development of epileptic symptoms due to excessive electrical or chemical stimulation to the brain. The experimental "kindling" process (Adamec & Stark-Adamec, 1983) will be described in greater detail later in chapter 13 when we discuss the possible physiological mechanisms that may underlie the development of MIND-like symptoms.

Thus far, we have discussed only case series of adult patients who have been treated with a mood-stabilizer followed traumatic brain injury. However, pediatric neuropsychologist M.A. Roberts and her colleagues reported on a series of 27 pediatric patients with multiple episodic symptoms who were given open trials on either carbamazepine or valproic acid (Roberts, Verduyn, Manshadi, & Hines, 1996). Of treated patients, 92% were judged to have exhibited moderate or substantial improvement following treatment. The authors concluded:

> Considered together, these findings suggest that dysfunctioning children and adolescents sustaining mild TBI suffer subclinical electrophysiological dysfunction . . . (p. 745)

To our knowledge, this represents the only systematic outcome data on a series of children and adolescents with significant symptoms of MIND.

When considered together, the results from case-series studies of open trials of treatment with either carbamazepine or valproic acid consistently have demonstrated that a majority of patients who report multiple intermittent symptoms following traumatic brain injury respond favorably to these two mood-stabilizing medications. In addition, Packard (2000) has demonstrated that valproic acid has efficacy in treating certain types of post-traumatic headaches. Although a comprehensive survey of the effectiveness of mood-stabilizing medications upon impulsive aggression is well beyond the scope of this book, it should be noted that anticonvulsant medications have frequently been prescribed for control of impulsive or irritable outbursts (e.g., Stanford et al., 2005). According to Stanford and his associates (Stanford, Anderson, Lake, & Baldridge, 2009):

> A review of the literature finds that AEDs [anti-epileptic drugs] . . . are effective in reducing the frequency and intensity of impulsive aggressive outbursts both when used as the primary agent of treatment and as an adjunct to ongoing pharmacotherapy. Strong evidence for efficacy in impulsive aggression exists from randomized controlled trials for most of the common AEDs (phenytoin, carbamazepine, oxcarbazepine, lamotrigine, valproate/divalproex sodium, topirimate). (p. 383)

In addition to the preceding review by Stanford et al. (2009), the interested reader also is referred to a recent review of pharmacological treatment of impulsive aggression in children and adolescents by Barzman & Findling (2008) and a detailed presentation of the neurobiology of impulsive aggression in general (Siever, 2008)—with or without clinical histories of head trauma.

Recent studies on the effectiveness of anticonvulsant mood stabilizers in treating major depressive disorder (regardless of history of head trauma) have been reviewed by Vigo & Baldessarini (2009). These authors concluded:

> Some of these trials, as well as 7 of lesser quality, suggest benefits of carbamazepine, lamotrigine, and valproate, mainly as adjuncts to ADs [antidepressant medications]. Another 20 anecdotes or small trials further suggest that these ACs [anticonvulsants] might be useful as AD adjuncts—specifically to treat irritability or agitation in MDD. (p. 231)

Consistent with the preceding conclusion, Pasquini et al. treated 35 patients with major depressive disorder and "substantial anger, irritability, or hostility" with open trials of the *combination* of an anticonvulsant mood-stabilizer *and* an SSRI antidepressant (Pasquini et al., 2007). On the basis of their promising results, they concluded:

> . . . we observed a remarkable improvement in most unipolar depressed outpatients with dysphoric mood treated with an SSRI and an anticonvulsant. The effectiveness of anticonvulsants might be linked to their actions on symptoms of aggression and behavioral activation. (p. 155)

We have mentioned explicitly the study of Pasquini et al. (2007) because: (1) it was not included in the review by Vigo & Baldessarini (2009); and (2) even though information regarding brain injury was lacking, the Pasquini study provides a model for using these two types of pharmacological agents to treat different aspects of impulsive aggression (Siever, 2008).

Case Studies

In the discipline of neuropsychiatry and the literature on traumatic brain injury, advances in assessment and treatment often begin modestly with the publication of single case studies. In Table 6–1, we provide a guide to some instructive case studies involving the treatment of MIND-like patients (particularly affective lability and anger/aggression) with anticonvulsant mood stabilizers. Because this information is primarily of importance to clinicians and researchers, we decided to summarize the most pertinent case-studies so that patients, their family members, and lay readers would not be burdened with excessive detail. Although these case studies have been selected for their individual heuristic value, it is evident from Table 6–1 that interest in the use of anticonvulsant medications as mood-stabilizing agents following brain injury and in the treatment of borderland conditions clearly accelerated in the decade between 1980 and 1990 (Post et al., 1998).

Summary

Although double-blind placebo-controlled studies and randomized controlled trials are lacking with regard to the treatment of MIND, clinical recommendations of prominent clinicians and evidence from a variety of other sources supports the use of mood-stabilizing medications for treating the intermittent symptoms of patients with traumatic brain injuries.

In the next chapter, we review some technical aspects of how physicians prescribe, monitor, and manage two such medications: carbamazepine and valproic acid.

Table 6-1. Selected Case Studies Relevant to the Pharmacological Treatment of MIND-like Patients

Authors	Year	N	Relevant Findings and Conclusions
Andy	1989	1	A woman developed "many diverse and unexplainable symptoms" over a 10-year period following serious head injury; she was treated successfully with electrical stimulation of the brain stem; this case suggests that some MIND-like patients may have occult, mid-brain lesions.
Barkai et al	2004	1	Successful treatment of MIND-like, episodic symptoms with valproic acid was associated with a "remarkable increase in frontal perfusion" following an episode of "mild" TBI with only "brief" loss of consciousness. There was remission of episodic symptoms at 3 months, but the patient was still unemployed. CT and MRI were both negative.
Blumer, Heilbronn, & Himmelhoch	1988	8	The authors present multiple case studies of successfully treated patients with "temporal lobe syndrome," focusing on indications for the use of carbamazepine.
Bouvy, van de Wetering, Meerwaldt, & Bruijn	1988	1	Eight months following a moderately severe TBI in a car accident, the patient suddenly developed psychosis due to an "organic brain syndrome;" EEG results were negative; the authors speculate that "kindling" may be involved in producing the delayed onset of symptoms.
Fincham, Yamada, Schottelius, Hayreh, & Damasio	1979	1	Damasio and his colleagues were the first to suggest that dichotic listening failure may be sensitive to underlying electrical dysfunction in a patient with atypical absence spells in the context of "normal behavior."

Authors	Year	N	Relevant Findings and Conclusions
Geracioti	1994	1	Valproic acid successful in treating "episodic explosiveness" due to brain injury, even though other mood abnormalities and psychotic features were absent; the author raises the possibility of a "subclinical seizure disorder."
Goetz	1987	1	The author reports a case of 19th century neurologist Charcot that demonstrated "bizarre ambulatory spells" and "complex interactions" with other people that were later unrecalled by the patient.
Goldstein	1984	1	Report of a single case of a military veteran with history of concussion in Vietnam effectively treated with mysoline for multiple, intermittent symptoms, headaches, and irritable outbursts; this case is fairly prototypic of a complex presentation that is fairly common among Vietnam veterans with histories of mild TBI.
Horne & Lindley	1995	3	Three patients with different brain-related etiologies were treated successfully with divalproex; aggressive behaviors and bouts of affective lability were reduced.
Jonas	1967a	1	The author, who in 1965 published a book on "subictal neurosis" (i.e., concept similar to MIND), draws attention to the use of anticonvulsants to treats "paroxysmal" headache that is not responsive to ergot medications; case-study use of phenytoin to treat headaches with mixed features of both migraine and epilepsy was successful.
Kemp	1992	1	Female patient with treatment-resistant depression and irritability successfully treated with valproic acid.

continues

Table 6–1. *continued*

Authors	Year	N	Relevant Findings and Conclusions
Kessler, Barklage, & Jefferson	1989	3	Jefferson and associates report on three patients with "mood disorder in the psycho-neurologic borderland" between epilepsy and atypical psychosis; all three patients responded to carbamazepine so favorably that previously prescribed neuroleptic medications could be discontinued; the authors hypothesis that "subictal activity in the limbic system" may be responsible for the patient's atypical clinical pictures.
Lewin & Sumners	1992	1	A case of episodic dyscontrol with violent outbursts and legal involvement following head injury in a traffic was treated successfully with carbamazepine; further outbursts subsided following treatment. EEG showed only an excess of theta activity.
Liebman & Rodriguez	2009	1	Case study of a patient with a conventional complex partial seizure disorder who subsequently developed nocturnal, MIND-like symptoms. The patient had been seizure-free for 3 years when this happened. This case suggests that the development of MIND-like symptoms may reflect a separate condition from conventional seizures with a distinct clinical presentation in its own right.
Mas, Prichep, & Alper	1993	1	Treatment-resistant depression is treated successfully with carbamazepine following head trauma; quantitative EEG exam was useful in detecting underlying electrical dysfunction; authors suggest there may be a neuro-electric subtype of treatment-resistant depression.

Authors	Year	N	Relevant Findings and Conclusions
McAllister	1985	5	Veteran patients with evidence of frontal lobe dysfunction and affective lability successfully treated with carbamazepine.
McElroy, Keck, Pope, & Hudson	1988	6	Pope and colleagues report on successful treatment using valproic acid of a series of cases with "rapid-cycling," treatment-resistant, bipolar disorder.
Monroe	1989	20	Of 20 patients with "episodic dyscontrol" syndrome who were treated with anticonvulsants, 16 (80%) were judged to manifest at least "moderate" improvement; 10 of these 16 showed "marked improvement" (50%); the author stresses importance of the theoretical construct "seizure threshold" when prescribing for such patients.
Neppe & Kaplan	1988	1	A provocative case study which suggests that some MIND patients may be withdrawn from anticonvulsant medication if they are treated acutely with carbamazepine.
Neppe, Bowman, & Sawchuk	1991	9	The authors present a series of cases of "atypical psychosis with episodic hostility" that responded favorably to treatment with carbamazepine.
Poprawski et al.	2007	1	This case illustrates how "multimodal imaging" can be used diagnostically in a complex patient with depression and violent behavior; the patient eventually was treated successfully with topiramate, an anticonvulsant.

continues

Table 6-1. *continued*

Authors	Year	N	Relevant Findings and Conclusions
Roberts et al.	1989	40	The authors demonstrate that MIND patients typically produced extremely elevated MMPI profiles and failed a dichotic word listening task.
Roberts	2008	1	Successful treatment of military veteran with divalproex and doxepine following blast-exposures in combat.
Roberts, Manshadi, Bushnell, & Hines	1995	1	14-year-old patient manifested persistent symptoms of MIND for 4 year post-TBI; was successfully treated with a combination of carbamazepine, verapimil, and fluoxetine; PET scan showed marked hypo-metabolism in both temporal lobes; this is the only published study of a MIND patient with functional neuro-imaging.
Ros	2004	1	Case report demonstrates that dysphoric attacks and chronic low-level depression may co-exist in the same patient; treatment with carbamazepine, clonazepam, and sertraline eliminated both types of dysphoric mood.
Stewart & Bartucci	1986	1	Successful treatment of atypical nocturnal spells and nightmares in PTSD patient using carbamazepine.
Stone, McDaniel, Hughes, & Hermann	1986	1	Unprovoked bouts of anger typically were preceded by "a funny feeling and buzzing in my head;" treatment of this case of Intermittent Explosive Disorder with carbamazepine was successful, but the patient's post-treatment MMPI profile continued to remain grossly elevated.

Authors	Year	N	Relevant Findings and Conclusions
Tunks & Dermer	1977	1	Early literature review and case-study on the effects of carbamazepine upon aggressive and sometimes violent behavior; the authors assert that carbamazepine has both anticonvulsant and "psychotropic" properties and that its use should be considered "in certain instances of dyscontrol, with or without clinical diagnosis of epilepsy."
Weiss & Spiegel	2008	1	An interesting case of partial motor seizures that apparently induced a transient amnestic syndrome.
Wieser, Hailermariam, Regard, & Landis	1992	4	Depth-electrodes studies (stereo-electroencephalography) showed that an entire hemisphere may be electrically dysfunctional with only subjective changes in behavior (i.e., unilateral limbic epileptic status).
Woodman & Noyes	1994	12	These cases with panic disorder were successfully treated with divalproex, indicating that valproic acid may have anti-anxiety properties, as well as being effective for managing impulsive anger and aggression
Yatham & McHale	1988	1	Carbamazepine treatment markedly reduced spells of aggressive behavior in a 18 year-old male; EEG was abnormal, but not clearly epileptiform.

References

Adamec, R. E., & Stark-Adamec, C. (1983). Limbic kindling and animal behavior—implications for human psychopathology associated with complex partial seizures. *Biological Psychiatry*, *18*, 269–293.

Anderson, R. J. (2008). Shell shock: An old injury with new weapons. *Molecular Interventions*, *8*, 204–218.

Andy, O. J. (1989). Post concussion syndrome: Brainstem seizures, a case report. *Clinical Electroencephalography*, *20*, 24–34.

Ashman, T. A., Cantor, J. B., Gordon, W. A., Spielman, L., Flanagan, S., Ginsberg, A., . . . & Greewald, B. (2009). A randomized controlled trial of sertraline for the treatment of depression in persons with traumatic brain injury. *Archives of Physical Medicine and Rehabilitaion*, *90*, 733–740.

Barkai, G., Goshen, E., Tzila Zwas, S., Dolberg, O. T., Pcik, C. G., Bonne, O., & Schreiber, S. (2004). Acetazolamide-enhanced neuroSPECT scan reveals functional impairment after minimal traumatic brain injury not otherwise discernable. *Psychiatry Research*, *132*, 279–283.

Barzman, D. H., & Findling, R. L. (2008). Pharmacological treatment of pathologic aggression in children. *International Review of Psychiatry*, *20*, 151–157.

Blumer, D. (2000). Dysphoric disorders and paroxysmal affects: Recognition and treatment of epilepsy-related psychiatric disorders. *Harvard Review of Psychiatry*, *8*, 8–17.

Blumer, D., Heilbronn, M., & Himmelhoch, J. (1988). Indications for carbamazepine in mental illness: Atypical psychiatric disorder or temporal lobe syndrome. *Comprehensive Psychiatry*, *29*, 108–122.

Blumer, D., Montouris, G., & Davies, K. (2004). The interictal dysphoric disorder: Recognition, pathogenesis, and treatment of the major psychiatric disorder of epilepsy. *Epilepsy and Behavior*, *5*, 826–840.

Bouvy, P. F., van de Wetering, B. J., Meerwaldt, J. D., & Bruijn, J. B. (1988). A case of organic brain syndrome following head injury successfully treated with carbamazepine. *Acta Psychiatrica Scandinavica, 77*, 361–363.

Fann, J. R., Hart, T., & Schomer, K. G. (2009). Treatment for depression after traumatic brain injury: A systematic review. *Journal of Neurotrauma, 26*, 2383–2402.

Fincham, R. W., Yamada, T., Schottelius, D. D., Hayreh, S. M., & Damasio, A. (1979). Electroencephalographic absence status with minimal behavior change. *Archives of Neurology, 36*, 176–178.

Fogel, B. S., Duffy, J., McNamara, M. E., & Salloway (1992). Skeptics and enthusiasts in neuropsychiatry. *Journal of Clinical Neuropsychiatry, 4*, 458–462.

Francisco, G. E., Walker, W. C., Zasler, N. D., & Bouffard, M. H. (2007). Pharmacological management of neurobehavioral sequelae of traumatic brain injury: A survey of current physiatric practice. *Brain Injury, 21*, 1007–1014.

Geracioti, T. D., Jr. (1994). Valproic acid treatment of episodic explosiveness related to brain injury. *Journal of Clinical Psychiatry, 55*, 416–417.

Goetz, C. G., (1987). Charcot at the Salpetriere: Ambulatory automatisms. *Neurology, 37*, 1084–1088.

Goldstein, G. C., (1984). Neuropsychological assessment of psychiatric patients. In G. Goldstein (Ed.), *Advances in clinical neuropsychology* (Vol. 1, pp. 59–75). New York, NY: Plenum Press.

Hachinski, V. (1990) Cognitive rehabilitation. *Archives of Neurology, 47*, 224.

Han, M. H., Craig, S. B., Rutner, D., Kapoor, N., Ciuffreda, K. J., & Suchoff, I. B. (2008). Medications prescribed to brain injury patients: A retrospective analysis. *Optometry, 79*, 252–258.

Hines, M., Swan, C., Roberts, R. J., & Varney, N. R. (1995). Characteristics and mechanisms of epilepsy spectrum disorder: An explanatory model. *Applied Neuropsychology, 2*, 1–6.

Horne, M., & Lindley, S. E. (1995). Divalproex sodium in the treatment of aggressive behavior and dysphoria in patients with organic brain syndromes. *Journal of Clinical Psychiatry, 56*, 430–431.

Jonas, A. D. (1967a). The distinction between paroxysmal and non-paroxysmal migraine. *Headache, 7*, 79–84.

Jonas, A. D. (1967b). The diagnostic and therapeutic use of diphenylhydantoin in the subictal state and non-epileptic dysphoria. *International Journal of Neuropsychiatry, 3(suppl.)*, 21–29.

Kemp L. I. (1992). Sodium valproate as an antidepressant. *British Journal of Psychiatry, 160*, 121–123.

Kessler, A. J., Barklage, N. E., & Jefferson, J. W. (1989). Mood disorders in the psychoneurologic borderland: Three cases of responsiveness to carbamazepine. *American Journal of Psychiatry, 146*, 81–83.

Kim, E., & Humaran, T. J. (2002). Divalproex in the management of neuropsychiatric complications of remote acquired brain injury. *Journal of Neuropsychiatry and Clinical Neuroscience, 14*, 202–205.

Lewin, J., & Sumners, D. (1992). Successful treatment of episodic dyscontrol with carbamazepine. *British Journal of Psychiatry, 161*, 261–262.

Liebman, R. F., & Rodriguez, A. J. (2009). A patient with epilepsy and new onset of nocturnal symptoms. *Review of Neurologic Disease, 6*, 37–38.

Lux, W. E. (2007). A neuropsychiatric perspective on traumatic brain injury. *Journal of Rehabilitation Research and Development, 44*, 951–962.

Mas, F., Prichep, L. S., & Alper. K. (1993). Treatment resistant depression in a case of minor head injury: An electrophysiological hypothesis. *Clinical Electroencephalography, 24*, 118–122.

McAllister, T. W. (1985). Carbamazepine in mixed frontal lobe and psychiatric disorders. *Journal of Clinical Psychiatry, 46*, 393–394.

McElroy, S. L., Keck, P. E., Pope, H. G., Jr., & Hudson, J. I. (1988). Valproate in the treatment of rapid-cycling bipolar disorder. *Journal of Clinical Psychopharmacology, 8*, 275–279.

Monroe, R. R. (1989). Dyscontrol syndrome: Long-term follow-up. *Comprehensive Psychiatry, 30*, 489–497.

Neppe, V. M., Bowman, B. R., & Sawchuk, K. S. (1991). Carbamazepine for atypical psychosis with episodic hostility. *Journal of Nervous and Mental Disease, 179*, 434–441.

Neppe, V. M., & Kaplan, C. (1988). Short-term treatment of atypical spells with carbamazepine. *Clinical Neuropharmacology, 11,* 287–289.

Neppe, V. M., & Tucker, G. J. (1994). Neuropsychiatric aspects of seizure disorders. In S. Yudofsky & S. Silver (Eds.), *The American Psychiatric Press textbook of neuropsychiatry* (pp. 397–425). Washington, DC: American Psychiatric Press.

Packard, R. C. (2000). Treatment of chronic daily headache with divalproex sodium. *Headache, 40,* 736–739.

Pasquini, M., Picardi, A., Speca, A., Orlandi, V., Tarsitani, L., Morosini, P., . . . & Biondi, M. (2007). Combining an SSRI with an anticonvulsant in depressed patients with dysphoric mood: An open study. *Clinical Practice of Epidemiology in Mental Health, 8,* 3–10.

Persinger, M. A. (2000). Subjective improvement following treatment with carbamazepine (Tegretol) for a subpopulation of patients with traumatic brain injuries. *Perceptual and Motor Skills, 90,* 37–40.

Poprawski, T. J., Pluzycaka, A. N., Park, Y., Chennamchetty, V. N., Halaris, A., Crayton, J. W., & Konopka, L. M. (2007). Multimodality imaging in a depressed patient with violent behavior and temporal lobe seizures. *Clinical EEG and Neuroscience, 38,* 175–179.

Post, R. M., Denicoff, K. D., Frye, M. A., Dunn, R. T., Leverich, G. S., Isuch, E., & Speer, A. (1998). A history of the use of anticonvulsants as mood stabilizers in the last two decades of the 20th century. *Neuropsychobiology, 38,* 152–166.

Roberts, M. A., Manshadi, F. F., Bushnell, D. L., & Hines, M. E. (1995). Neurobehavioral dysfunction following mild traumatic injury in childhood: A case report with positive findings on positron emission tomography. *Brain Injury, 9,* 427–436.

Roberts, M. A., Verduyn, W. H., Manshadi, F. F., & Hines, M. E. (1996). Episodic symptoms in dysfunctioning children and adolescents following mild and severe traumatic brain injury. *Brain Injury, 10,* 739–747.

Roberts, R. J. (2009, December-January). Impact on the brain. *Scientific American Mind,* 50–57.

Roberts, R. J., Paulsen, J. S., Marchman, J. N., & Varney, N. R. (1989). MMPI profiles of patients who endorse multiple partial seizure symptoms. *Neuropsychology, 2,* 183–198.

Roberts, R. J., Varney, N. R., Paulsen, J. S., & Richardson, E. D. (1990). Dichotic listening and complex partial seizures. *Journal of Clinical and Experimental Neuropsychology, 12,* 448–458.

Ros, L. T. (2004). A case of "double" depression under outpatient treatment conditions. *World Journal of Biological Psychiatry, 5,* 161–163.

Siever, L. J. (2008). Neurobiology of aggression and violence. *American Journal of Psychiatry, 165,* 429–442.

Silver J. M., McAllister, T. W., & Arcinegas, D. B. (2009). Depression and cognitive complaints following mild traumatic brain injury. *American Journal of Psychiatry, 166,* 653–661.

Shapiro, F. (2001). *Eye movement desensitization and reprocessing (EMDR).* New York, NY: Guilford Press.

Stanford, M. S., Anderson, N. E., Lake, S. L., & Baldridge, R. M. Pharmacologic treatment of impulsive aggression with antiepileptic drugs. (2009). *Current Treatment Options in Neurology, 11,* 383–390.

Stanford, M. S., Helfritz, L. E., Conklin, S. M., Villemarte-Pittman, N. R., Greve, K. W., Adams, D., & Houston, R. J. (2005). A comparison of anticonvulsants in the treatment of impulsive aggression. *Experimental and Clinical Psychopharmacology, 13,* 72–77.

Stapert, S. Z. (2009). The post-concussion syndrome: Understanding and treating a disease process. *Tijdschr Psychiatry, 51,* 107–116.

Stewart, J. T., & Bartucci, R. J. (1986). Post-traumatic stress disorder and partial complex seizures. *American Journal of Psychiatry, 143,* 113–114.

Stone, J. L., McDaniel, K. D., Hughes, J. R., & Hermann, B. P. (1986). Episodic dyscontrol disorder and paroxysmal EEG abnormalities: Successful treatment and carbamazepine. *Biological Psychiatry, 21,* 208–212.

Taylor, M. A. (1999). *Fundamentals of clinical neuropsychiatry.* New York, NY: Oxford University Press.

Tierney, J. G., & Fogel, B. S. (1995). Neuropsychiatric sequelae of mild traumatic brain injury. In A. Stoudamire & B. S. Fogel (Eds.), Medical-psychiatric practice (Vol. 3, 307–380). Washington, DC: American Psychiatric Press.

Tucker, G. J. (1998). Seizure disorders presenting with psychiatric symptomatology. *Psychiatric Clinics of North America*, *21*, 625–635.

Tucker, G. J., Price, T. R. P., Johnson, V. B., & McAllister, T. (1986). Phenomenology of temporal lobe dysfunction: A link to atypical psychosis—a series of cases. *Journal of Nervous and Mental Disease*, *174*, 348–356.

Tunks, E. R., & Dermer, S. W. (1977). Carbamazepine in the dyscontrol syndrome associated with limbic system dysfunction. *Journal of Nervous and Mental Disease*, *164*, 56–63.

Varney, N. R., Garvey, M., Campbell, D., Cook, B., & Roberts, R. J. (1993). Identification of treatment-resistant depressives who respond favorably to carbamazepine. *Annals of Clinical Psychiatry*, *5*, 117–122.

Verduyn, W. H., Hilt, J., Roberts, M. A., & Roberts, R. J. (1992). Multiple partial seizure-like symptoms following "minor" head injury. *Brain Injury*, *6*, 245–260.

Vigo, D. V., & Baldessarini, R. J. (2009). Anticonvulsants in the treatment of major depressive disorder: an overview. *Harvard Review of Psychiatry*, *17*, 231–241.

Weiss, G. M., & Spiegel, D. R. (2008). Transient amnestic syndrome in the setting of recurrent partial elementary seizures. *Journal of Neuropsychiatry and Clinical Neuroscience*, *20*, 115–116.

Wieser, H. G., Hailermariam, M., Regard, M., & Landis, T. (1992). Unilateral limbic & epileptic status activity: Stereo EEG, behavioral, and cognitive data. *Epilepsia*, *26*, 19–29.

Woodman, C. L., & Noyes, R., Jr. (1994). Panic disorder: Treatment with valproate. *Journal of Clinical Psychiatry*, *55*, 134–136.

Wroblewski, B. A., Joseph, A. B., Kupfer, J., & Kalliel, K. (1997). Effectiveness of valproic acid on destructive and aggressive behaviors in patients with acquired brain injury. *Brain Injury*, *11*, 37–47.

Yasseen, B., Colantonio, A., & Ratcliff, G. (2008). Prescription medication use in persons many years following traumatic brain injury. *Brain Injury, 22,* 752–757.

Yatham, L. N. & McHale, P. A. (1988). Carbamazepine in the treatment of aggression: a case report and review of the literature. *Acta Psychiatrica Scandinavica, 78,* 188–190.

Zappala, G., & Cameron, J. S. (1990). Subictal and interictal temporal lobe phenomena in traumatic brain injury: Treatment with carbamazepine. *Advances in Brain Injury Rehabilitation, 1,* 3–4.

7

Mood-Stabilizing Medications with Anticonvulsant Properties

Perhaps most crucial to this diagnosis is the episodic nature and intensity of the pathology with apparent rapid return to normality. The clinicians observing such fluctuations should be alerted to think of these conditions. Such careful diagnostic evaluation is of obvious importance in patients such as these in whom specific drug treatment is both indicated and likely to provide benefit with respect to the behavioral pathology in question.

—G. Tucker, T. Price, V. Johnson, & T. McAllister (1986, p.354)

Introduction

This chapter reviews some practical aspects of prescribing two anticonvulsant mood stabilizers, carbamazepine (also known as Tegretol) and valproic acid (also known as sodium valproate,

Depakene, Depakote, and Divalproex). These two medications are most frequently used for treating the intermittent symptoms and emotional lability associated with MIND following blunt-force head trauma. Although this information has been reviewed by a board-certified psychiatrist, William Sheehan, M.D., and documented with references to primary sources from medical journals, the first two authors reaffirm that they themselves do *not* prescribe medications. Nor do they claim any specific expertise in psychopharmacology or the practice of neuropsychiatric medicine or epileptology beyond that afforded by their research interests.

We explicitly caution that individual patients reading this material should *not* take independent action in discontinuing and altering the dosage of *any* currently prescribed medication without first consulting their prescribing physician or care provider. Similarly, lay readers absolutely should *refrain* from experimenting with medications that have been prescribed for relatives or friends in hopes of treating themselves or their significant others. If readers have medical questions based upon material presented in this book, they should address such questions to their physicians or other medical care providers.

With medications used by psychiatrists and neurologists to treat disorders of the brain, successful treatment generally seeks to maximize the degree of symptomatic relief (i.e., the intended therapeutic effect) while minimizing unwanted side effects. These generic goals certainly apply to the use of both antidepressant and anticonvulsant medications following traumatic brain injury. Generally speaking, physicians aim to use the fewest medications possible and the lowest dosages of each individual medication to treat a given condition, such as MIND, following TBI in order to minimize the risk of unwanted side effects. Furthermore, some injured brains may develop marked sensitivities to certain prescription medications, so the adage, "*Start low and go slow,*" frequently applies to adjusting the dosage of psychoactive medications used to treat individuals who have sustained TBI (Lee, Lyketsos, & Rao, 2003).

Another important treatment issue is the concept of what constitutes "an adequate trial" of a particular medication. This phrase means giving a prescribed medication *sufficient time at a reasonable dosage* (or sufficient concentration in the bloodstream) to produce the intended therapeutic effects. Both anticonvulsant mood stabilizers and antidepressant medications typically need to build up over time in the bloodstream in order be effective. In the majority of cases, possible side effects will not be noticeable or minor during such a therapeutic trial. And if minor side effects are noticed by the patient, many of them tend to decrease or disappear entirely as the body adjusts to metabolizing a new medication.

Physicians usually need to conduct some simple blood tests before treating with either carbamazepine or valproic acid in order to assess a patient's liver function. Occasional blood tests also may be needed periodically during treatment to monitor liver functions on an ongoing basis, aspects of blood chemistry, or to document blood levels of a mood-stabilizing medication. In addition, periodic appointments with the prescribing care provider are necessary to monitor possible interactions between medications and to augment partial treatment response, if need be. The treating care provider may wish to re-administer part or all of the Iowa Interview to document that the frequencies of certain intermittent symptoms (such as target symptoms) have declined after favorable response to treatment has been established on general clinical grounds.

Although no hard and fast rules exist, the intermittent symptoms of MIND tend to respond to successful treatment and decrease in a fairly orderly progression. With most successfully treated cases of MIND we have observed, psycho-sensory illusions and unformed hallucinations appear to respond earliest, followed by untriggered emotional spells of dysphoric mood, panic, and irritability. It is most often the intermittent cognitive symptoms, such as brief memory lapses, confusional spells, and word-finding lapses, which prove to be most resistant to pharmacological treatment. At the present time, we are unsure why this appears to be the case.

Frequent sick headaches and cephalic pain may either respond very favorably to preventive treatment with a mood stabilizer (particularly valproic acid, according to Packard [2000]); however, post-traumatic headaches may require the addition of other anti-headache medication after a severe headache has started acutely (Silberstein, 2009). Intermittent sleep-related symptoms also generally improve, unless there is a completely different comorbid sleep disorder that requires additional assessment and treatment (e.g., sleep apnea syndrome). An adequate therapeutic trial of either mood stabilizer discussed in this chapter may, thus, take a full 6 to 10 weeks before maximum therapeutic benefit (or lack thereof) has been established.

Strict compliance with treatment instructions (i.e., taking one's medication on a regular schedule as instructed by the prescribing care provider) promotes achieving a favorable response to treatment as quickly as possible. If the particular patient being treated has discrete memory lapses, problems with prospective memory function (i.e., remembering when to take action at the time the action is needed), or personal disorganization (often associated with prefrontal damage or dysfunction), then it may well be necessary to put a more reliable person (such as a family member, significant other, or visiting nurse) in control of medication to establish compliance until the taking of medication becomes part of one's daily routine.

Carbamazepine

For treating conventional seizure disorders, this medication usually is prescribed 2 or 3 times per day at an eventual level of between 600 and 1200 mg. for each dose. This typically results in a therapeutic plasma level of between 4 to 12 micrograms/milliliter (Devinsky, 2003). However, treating prescribers almost always start with a much smaller dose. Then, they will raise the dosage slowly, in order to minimize possible minor side-effects. Although we cannot present systematic data at this time, we have observed that successful treatment of MIND symptoms often occurs at the lower end of the therapeutic range when carbamazepine is used to treat conventional seizure disorders.

Thus, a patient with MIND may exhibit a quite satisfactory response with a blood level in the range of 4 to 8 micrograms/milliliter.

Common side effects of carbamazepine may include sedation, headache, blurred or double vision, gastrointestinal symptoms, rash, ataxia (reduced motor coordination and unsteady gait), tremor, or neutropenia (a decrease in the number of neutrophils, a type of white blood cell). Medically serious adverse reactions include osteopenia (lowered bone density, a precursor to possible osteoporosis), hyponatremia (abnormally low concentration of sodium in the plasma of the blood), cardiac arrhythmias, Stevens-Johnson syndrome (an infrequent but potentially life-threatening reaction characterized by fever and flu-like symptoms followed by a severe, blistering rash on the skin and/or mucous membranes), hematologic toxicity (reduction of clotting factors in the blood), and hepatic toxicity (being poisonous to, or destructive of, liver cells). Longitudinal study of patients who have been prescribed anticonvulsant medication for psychiatric reasons has demonstrated that consistent anticonvulsant treatment was associated with decreased risk of completed suicide (Smith, Sondergard, Lopez, Anderson, & Kessing, 2009); however, intentional overdose using anticonvulsant medications, including carbamazepine, can have serious medical consequences (Graudins, Peden, & Dowsett, 2002; Nixon, Doak, Crozier, Crooks, & Waring, 2009; Sethna, Solomon, Cedarbaum, & Kutt, 1989).

Blood levels of carbamazepine may fall acutely with diarrhea due to flu or excessive perspiration due to extremely hot weather (Parnas, Flachs, Gram, & Wurtz-Jorgensen, 1978) to the point where certain patients (or their significant others) may notice a transient return or intensification of some intermittent symptoms (e.g., more memory lapses, resumption of rage outbursts, etc.). Should this happen, the prescribing care provider should be contacted. Also, carbamazepine may lower the effectiveness of some birth control pills; thus, the method of contraception employed is of concern for women of child-bearing age (Crawford, 2009; Schindlbeck, Janni, & Friese, 2006). The use of anticonvulsant medications during pregnancy has been the subject of several recent reviews (Crawford, 2009; Harden et al., 2009; Meador et al., 2009). The potential risks of taking carbamazepine during pregnancy should be discussed with the patient, and this discussion should be documented explicitly in the medical record (James, Barnes, Lelliott, Taylor, & Paton, 2007).

Care should be taken to store carbamazepine in a light-blocking container in places with low humidity because contact with water or extremely humid air (e.g., due to bathrooms without adequate ventilation) can decrease markedly the effectiveness of carbamazepine (Bell, Crawford, & Shiu, 1993; Wang, Shiu, Ong-Chen, Viswanathan, & Skelly 1993). For selected patients, brand-name Tegretol has been observed to be more effective than generic carbamazepine (Borgheini, 2003). Carbamazepine also is marketed as Carbatrol in the form of extended-release capsules (Hogan, Garnett, Thadani, & Carbatrol Study Group, 2003). Prior to being prescribed carbamazepine or Tegretol, physicians should assess possible drug-drug interactions between this mood stabilizer and other prescription medications, particularly with other anticonvulsants. Although somewhat dated, an article by Neppe, Tucker, & Wilensky (1988) provides a very accessible review of the technical fundamentals of prescribing carbamazepine in neuropsychiatric practice.

In addition to treating epileptic disorders, carbamazepine also has been shown to be of value in treating bipolar affective disorder (e.g., Rapoport, Basselin, Kim, & Rao, 2009) and chronic neuropathic pain (Dobecki, Schoket, & Wallace, 2006). It also may be used to treat patients with histories of impulsive aggression or dyscontrol syndromes (Pae, 2008; Stanford et al., 2005) and treatment-refractory depression (Vigo & Baldessarini, 2009).

Valproic Acid

For treating conventional forms of epilepsy, this prescription medication usually is prescribed two or three times per day in dosages ranging from 1000 to 3000 mg. The therapeutic range of blood plasma levels for treating seizures typically varies from

50 to 120 micrograms per milliliter. However, as with prescribing carbamazepine, care providers typically will begin to prescribe valproic acid at a much lower dosage and then gradually raise the dosage over time. Although we lack systematic data, positive clinical response to treating symptoms of MIND with valproic acid can be observed at the lower end of the therapeutic range for treating conventional seizures (e.g., 50 to 80 micrograms per milliliter).

Possible side effects of valproic acid include nausea, vomiting, sedation, weight gain, hair loss, tremor, thrombocytopenia (presence of a reduced number of platelets in the blood), excessive bruising, irregular menses, and hyperammonemia (i.e., a metabolic disturbance defined by the presence of excessive ammonia in the bloodstream) (Devinsky, 2003). Potentially severe side effects include polycystic ovarian syndrome (cysts in the ovaries), osteopenia, encephalopathy (confusion compromising brain function), pedal edema (swelling of the lower legs or ankles), liver failure, and pancreatitis (inflammation of the pancreas). Valproic acid has been found to decrease suicidal potential in bipolar psychiatric patients with good compliance (Yerevanian, Koek, & Mintz, 2007). However, as also is true for carbamazepine, intentional overdose with valproic acid can result in serious medical consequences (Hurdle & Moss, 2009; Lokan & Dinan, 1988; Sztajnkrycer, 2002; Willimowska, Florek, & Peikoszewski, 2006). Some experts feel that the use of valproic acid is associated with a reduced side-effect profile compared to that associated with prescription of carbamazepine.

Technical aspects of prescribing valproic acid for neuropsychiatric patients have been summarized by a number of clinicians (Bowden, 2007; Bowden, 2009; Centorrino et al., 2003; Davis, Ryan, Adinoff, & Petty, 2000; Fleming & Chetty, 2006; Haddad, Das, Ashfaq, & Wieck, 2009; Keck & McElroy, 2002; Kim & Humaran, 2002). Valproic acid is available in both extended-release and delayed release formulations. Evidence shows that taking valproic acid during pregnancy is associated with increased risk of serious birth defects, and these risks should be taken into consideration and openly discussed with women of child-bearing age (Aisdorf & Wyszynski, 2005; Ornoy, 2009; Tomson & Battino, 2009). Valproic acid does not appear to alter the effectiveness of commonly used birth control preparations (Crawford, 2009), however. Evidence of possible drug-drug interactions with other anticonvulsants and psychotropic medications has been reported. However, valproic acid appears to be relatively free of deleterious cognitive effects when compared to most other anticonvulsants used to treat seizures in frankly epileptic patients (Dikmen, Machamer, Winn, Anderson, & Temkin, 2000).

In addition to being a first-line anticonvulsant medication, valproic acid also has been used to treat bipolar disorder, agitation in the context of dementia or severe brain injury, preventive treatment of migraine headaches, aggressive behaviors in youths, and impulsivity in the context of certain personality disorders (Bowden, 2007; Davis, Ryan, Adinoff, & Petty, 2000; Haddad, Das, Asfaq, & Wieck, 2009; Kim & Humaran, 2002). Technical aspects of prescribing valproic acid in adult neuropsychiatry have been summarized by Bowden (2007). Various technical aspects of prescribing valproic acid for children and adolescents also have been discussed recently by numerous authors (e.g., Apostol et al., 2009; Lenz, Eleterman, Robieson, Vigma, & Satarelli, 2009; Verrotto, la Torre, Trotta, Mohn, & Chiarelli, 2009; Wagner et al., 2009),

Treatment Alternatives

When a head-injured patient with significant symptoms of MIND on the Iowa Interview has failed to tolerate an adequate, clinical trial of either carbamazepine or valproic acid, or treatment has not produced a favorable outcome, instituting an empirical trial of the other mood stabilizer is a reasonable course of action. However, in our experience, a number of initial treatment failures can be explained by poor compliance or patient misconceptions as to how they should be taking their medication. If a patient has not responded clinically, *always remember to check compliance.* (Similarly, if a patient who has been doing well suddenly becomes more dysfunctional, *always remember to check compliance.*) Routinely checking blood levels also may promote better compliance in some patients with questionable compliance (Fleming & Chetty, 2006).

Should a patient fail to respond favorably to adequate trials of carbamazepine *and* valproic acid, the prescribing clinician would do well to step back and reconsider the working diagnosis. As discussed elsewhere in this book, extremely dissociative patients with histories of severe child abuse occasionally do produce elevated scores on the Iowa Interview on the basis of abrupt shifts in ego-states, rather than on the basis of subclinical electrophysiological dysfunction. Re-interviewing an initially nonresponsive patient for a history of possible psychological trauma, obtaining permission to contact collateral informants, or requesting a second opinion from a clinician specializing in dissociative phenomena are all worthwhile alternatives to consider when a patient has failed to improve on adequate therapeutic trials of both carbamazepine and valproic acid.

When a patient has failed to tolerate either carbamazepine or valproic acid due to unwanted side effects, other potentially useful pharmacological agents with mood-stabilizing properties include oxcarbazepine, phenytoin, lamotrigine, and longer-acting benzodiazepines, such as clonazepam. Benzodiazepine antianxiety agents generally are contraindicated in patients with traumatic brain injury due to producing excessive sedation. However, we have observed patients with MIND who have responded favorably to clonazepam in the rare circumstance of having developed side effects to all other anticonvulsant mood stabilizers tried.

SSRI antidepressants often are useful adjuncts to primary treatment of MIND with one anticonvulsant mood stabilizer or another, especially when emotional symptoms such as sadness, irritability, or general emotional lability persist. Contrary to clinical lore of yester-year, recent evidence suggests that SSRI medications have mildly *anticonvulsive properties* at the dosages used to treat major depressive disorder (Dailey & Naritoku, 1996; Jobe, 2004).

Mood stabilizers (such as carbamazepine and valproic acid) and SSRI antidepressant medications can both reduce impulsive behavior; however, their mechanisms of action upon brain neurotransmitters are likely to be quite different (Siever, 2008). Thus, the combination of a mood stabilizer and an SSRI antidepressant (Gyulai et al., 2003) may prove to be a rational consideration, if residual moodiness and irritability persist in patients with MIND following the partially successful use of a mood stabilizer (Pasquini et al., 2007).

Should MIND patients continue to complain of increased mental fatigue or slowed mental processing speed following TBI (despite good clinical response to a mood stabilizer), a trial of a low-dose stimulant medication occasionally proves helpful. The effects of methylphenidate in moderate-to-severe TBI were studied in a rigorously controlled double-blind study by Willmott & Ponsford (2009). Their patients demonstrated significantly enhanced processing speed after treatment during the inpatient rehabilitation phase following TBI. These authors also found that the use of methylphenidate was relatively safe and free of adverse side effects (Willmott, Ponsford, Oliver, & Ponsford, 2009). The findings of Willmott and colleagues were similar to the conclusions of Siddall (2005), who had reviewed the earlier literature and concluded that methylphenidate can improve processing speed, attention and concentration, and memory function. Gucuyener and colleagues (2003) found that use of methylphenidate in children with conventional epilepsy did not lead to an increased frequency of seizures; furthermore, any side effects of this stimulant were observed to be "mild and transient" (Gucuyener et al., 2003).

In general, when prescribing medications for patients with mild TBI, it is preferable to avoid drugs with strong anticholinergic effects and sedative effects (with the occasional exception of enhancing sleep-onset at bedtime). It also is best to avoid prescribing medications such as buproprion (Wellbutrin) that are known to lower seizure threshold (i.e., medications that would make having a conventional epileptic seizure more likely to occur).

Integrating Pharmacotherapy with Behavioral Interventions

Not every symptom or life problem associated with MIND can be addressed completely simply by taking prescribed medications. With adults, often personal adjustment, vocational, and family issues need to be addressed behaviorally following TBI. With children and adolescents, frequently educational and behavioral issues need to be addressed. In our experiences, after the identified patient has been optimally treated in a pharmacological sense, it usually becomes easier for patients to engage in counseling or psycho-educational and behavioral interventions in order to address unresolved issues. This observation is quite similar to the clinical conclusions of A.D. Jonas (1965) several decades ago. Fortunately, clinical neuropsychologists and rehabilitation psychologists (e.g., Allen, 2007; McCrea, 2008; Snell, Surgenor, Hay-Smith, & Siegert, 2009) have begun to devote increased attention to delivering behavioral services to patients and their families in conjunction with pharmacologic treatment.

Because no two traumatic brain injuries are exactly alike, the focus of counseling and other behavioral interventions needs to be adapted to the specific needs of each individual patient and family. Although "manualized" approaches to group psycho-educational interventions can be helpful in discerning issues for later individualized interventions, cookie cutter approaches to treatment (i.e., where it is assumed that the patient automatically fits the therapy that the counselor is prepared to vend) may overlook the specific needs of a given patient of family. This is particularly true when there are pre-existing conditions (e.g., PTSD from child abuse, combat, or sexual trauma in adulthood) or ongoing clinical issues (e.g., marital discord, substance abuse, oppositional/defiant disorder in childhood) that have been exacerbated following TBI. If multiple care providers or specialists are treating different aspects of the postacute, clinical picture, it is important that different aspects of treatment be coordinated (Batten & Pollack, 2008). With adult MIND patients, it is crucial that potential obstacles to return to work (such as difficulties with executive function) be investigated early on in the rehabilitation process to maximize the likelihood of success (Shames, Treger, Ring, & Giaquinto, 2007). Likewise, if orthopedic injuries were incurred at the same time, chronic pain complaints need to be addressed (Nampiaparampil, 2008). The effects of possible financial stress (and the potential for financial mismanagement if a given brain-injured patient in inappropriately managing his or her funds) also may need to be confronted (Spinella, Yang, & Lester, 2004; Spinella, Yang, & Lester, 2007). In short, much behavioral work often needs to be accomplished after the optimal effects of medication have been established.

A major point to be recognized, however, is that *behavioral interventions are more likely to be accepted after the symptoms of MIND have been treated successfully pharmacologically.* Swallowing "pills without skills"—or trying to teach "skills without pills"—either alternative in isolation usually proves less effective in helping MIND patients than does addressing both domains of care in a logical and well-timed sequence.

In the next two chapters, we discuss a potential cause of MIND that is even *more controversial* than blunt-force trauma: blast-exposure from explosions in combat.

References

Allen, E. A. (2007). Interventions for postconcussion syndrome. *Trauma, 9,* 181–187.

Alsdorf, R., & Wyszynski, D. F. (2005). Teratogenicity of sodium valproate. *Expert Opinion in Drug Safety, 4,* 345–353.

Apostol, G., Lewis, D. W., Laforet, G. A., Robieson, W. Z., Fugate, J. M., Abi-Saab, W. M., & Saltarelli, M. D. (2009). Divalproex sodium extended-release for the prophylaxis of migraine headache in adolescents: Results of a stand-alone, long-term open-label safety study. *Headache, 49,* 45–53.

Batten, S. V., & Pollack, S. J. (2008). Integrative outpatient treatment for returning service members. *Journal of Clinical Psychology, 64,* 928–939.

Bell, W. L., Crawford, I. L., & Shiu, G. K. (1993). Reduced bio-availability of moisture-exposed carbamazepine resulting in status epilepticus. *Epilepsia, 34,* 1102–1104.

Borgheini, G. (2003). The bioequivalence and therapeutic efficacy of generic versus brand-name psychoactive drugs. *Clinical Therapeutics, 25,* 1578–1592.

Bowden, C. L (2007) Spectrum of effectiveness of valproate in neuropsychiatry. *Expert Review of Neurotherapeutics, 7,* 9–16.

Bowden, C. L. (2009). Anticonvulsants in bipolar disorders: Current research and practice and future directions. *Bipolar Disorders, 11 (Suppl. 2),* 20–33.

Centorrino, F., Kelleher, J. P., Berry, J. M., Salvaltore, P., Eakin, M., Fogarty, K. V., . . . & Baldessarini, R. J. (2003). Pilot comparison of extended-release and standard preparations of divalproex sodium in patients with bipolar and schizoaffective disorders. *American Journal of Psychiatry, 160,* 1348–1350.

Crawford, P. M., (2009). Managing epilepsy in women of child-bearing age. *Drug Safety, 32,* 293–307.

Dailey, J. W., & Naritou, D. K. (1996). Antidepressants and seizures: Clinical anecdotes overshadow neuroscience. *Biochemical Pharmacology, 8,* 1323–1329.

Davis, L. L., Ryan, W., Adinoff, B., & Petty, F. (2000). Comprehensive review of the psychiatric uses of valproate. *Journal of Clinical Psychopharmacology, 20,* 1S–17S.

Devinsky, O. (2003). A 48-year-old man with temporal lobe epilepsy and psychiatric illness. *Journal of the American Medical Association, 290,* 381–392.

Dikmen, S. S., Machamer, J. E., Winn, H. R., Anderson, G. D., & Temkin, N. R. (2000). Neuropsychological effects of valproate in traumatic brain injury: A randomized trial. *Neurology, 22,* 895–902.

Dobecki, D. A., Schoket, S. M., & Wallace, M. S. (2006). Update on pharmacotherapy guidelines for the treatment of neuropathic pain. *Current Pain and Headache Report, 10,* 185–190.

Fleming, J., & Chetty, M. (2006). Therapeutic monitoring of valproate in psychiatry: How far have we progressed? *Clinical Neuropharmacology, 29,* 350–360.

Graudins, A., Peden, G., & Dowsett, R. P. (2002). Massive overdose with controlled-release carbamazepine resulting in delay peak serum concentrations and life-threatening toxicity. *Emergency Medicine* (Fremantle), *14*, 89–94.

Gucuyener, K., Erdemoglu, A. K., Senol, S., Serdaroglu, A., Sovsal, S., & Kockar, A. I., (2003). Use of methylphenidate for attention deficit hyperactivity disorder in patients with epilepsy or electroencephalographic abnormalities. *Journal of Child Neurology, 18*, 109–112.

Gyulia, L., Bowden, C. L., McElroy, S. L., Calabrese, J. R., Petty, F., Swann, A. C., . . . Wozniak, P. J. (2003). Maintenance efficacy of divalproex in the prevention of bipolar depression. *Neuropsychopharmacology, 28*, 1374–1382.

Haddad, P. M., Das, A., Ashfaq, M., & Wieck, A. (2009). A review of valproate in psychiatric practice. *Expert Opinion in Drug Metabolism and Toxicology, 5*, 539–551.

Harden, C. L., Pennell, P. B., Koppel, B. S., Hovinga, C. A., Gidal, B., Meador, K. J., . . . LeGuen, C. (2009). Practice parameter update: Management issues for women with epilepsy—focus on pregnancy (an evidence-based review): Vitamin K, folic acid, blood levels, and breastfeeding: Report of the Quality Standards Subcommittee and Therapeutics and Technology Assessment Subcommittee of the American Academy of Neurology and American Epilepsy Society. *Neurology, 73*, 142–149.

Hogan, R. E., Garnett, W. R., Thadani, V. M., & Carbatrol Study Group. (2003). Tolerability and effects on quality of life of twice-daily extended-release carbamazepine in adults with seizure disorder: An open-label, 12–36-month continuation study. *Clinical Therapeutics, 25*, 2586–2596.

Hurdle, A. C., & Moss, R. D. (2009). Unrecognized valproic acid intoxication. *American Journal of Emergency Medicine, 27*, e1–e2.

James, L., Barnes, T. R., Lelliot, P., Taylor, D., & Paton, C. (2007). Informing patients of the teratogenic potential of mood stabilizing drugs: A case review of the practice of psychiatrists. *Journal of Psychopharmacology, 21*, 815–819.

Jobe, P. C. (2004). Affective disorder and epilepsy comorbidity: Implications for development or treatments, preventions and diagnostic approaches. *Clinical EEG and Neurosicence, 35*, 53–68.

Jonas, A. D. (1965). *Ictal and subictal neurosis.* Springfield, IL.: C.C. Thomas.

Keck, P. E., Jr., & McElroy, S. L. (2002). Carbamazepine and valproate in the maintenance treatment of bipolar disorder. *Journal of Clinical Psychiatry, 63*(Suppl. 10), 13–17.

Kim, E., & Humaran, T. J. (2002). Divalproex in the management of neuropsychiatric complications of remote acquired brain injury. *Journal of Neuropsychiatry and Clinical Neuroscience, 14*, 202–205.

Lee, H. B., Lyketsos, C. G., & Rao, V. (2003). Pharmacological management of the psychiatric aspects of traumatic brain injury. *International Review of Psychiatry, 15*, 359–370.

Lenz, R. A., Eleterman, R. D., Robieson, W. Z., Vigna, N. V., & Saltarelli, M. D. Divalproex sodium in children with partial seizures: 12-month safety study. *Pediatric Neurology, 41*, 101–110.

Lokan, R. J., & Dinan, A. C. An apparent fatal valproic acid poisoning. *Journal of Analytic Toxicology, 12*, 35–37.

McCrea, M. A. (2008). *Mild traumatic brain injury and postconcussion syndrome: The new evidence base for diagnosis and treatment.* New York, NY: Oxford University Press.

Meador, K. J., Penovich, P., Baker, G. A., Pennell, P. B., Bromfield, E., Pack, A., . . . & NEAD Study Group. (2009). Antiepileptic drug use in women of childbearing age. *Epilepsy and Behavior, 15*, 339–343.

Nampiaparampil, D. E. (2008). Prevalence of chronic pain after traumatic brain injury: A systematic review. *Journal of the American Medical Association, 300*, 711–719.

Neppe, V. M., Doak, M. W., Crozier, H., Crooks, D. P., & Waring, W. S. (1988). Fundamentals of carbamazepine use in neuropsychiatry. *Journal of Clinical Psychiatry, 49*, S4–S6.

Nixon, A. C., Doak, M. W., Crozier, H., Crooks, D. P., & Waring, W. S. (2009). Patterns of antiepeileptic drug overdose differ between men and women: Admissions to the Edinburgh Poisons Unit, 2000–2007. *Quarterly Journal of Medicine, 102*, 51–56.

Ornoy, A. (2009). Valproic acid in pregnancy: How much are we endangering the embryo and fetus? *Reproductive Toxicology, 28*, 1–10.

Packard, R. C. (2000). Treatment of chronic daily headache with divalproex sodium. *Headache, 40*, 736–739.

Pae, C. U. (2008). Effectiveness of carbamazepine for benzodiazepine-resistant impulsive aggression in a patient with frontal infarctions. *Psychiatry and Clinical Neuroscience, 62*, 483.

Parnas, J., Flachs, H., Gram, L., & Wurtz-Jogensen, A. (1978). Execretion of antiepileptic drugs in sweat. *Acta Neurologica Scandinavica, 58*, 197–204.

Pasquini, M., Picardi, A., Speca, A., Orlandi, V., Tarsitani, L., Morosini, P., . . .Biondi, M. (2007). Combining an SSRI with an anticonvulsant in depressed patients with dysphoric mood: An open study. *Clinical Practice of Epidemiology in Mental Health, 8*, 3–10.

Rapoport, S. I., Basselin, M., Kim, H. W., & Rao, J. S. (2009). Bipolar disorder and mechanisms of action of mood stabilizers. *Brain Research Review, 61*, 185–209.

Schindlbeck, C., Janni, W, & Friese, K. (2006). Failure of Implanon contraception in a patient taking carbamazepine for epilepsy. *Archives of Gynecology and Obstetrics, 272*, 255–256.

Sethna, M., Solomon, G., Cedarbaum, J., & Kutt, H. (1989). Successful treatment of massive carbamazepine overdose. *Epilepsia, 30*, 71–73.

Siddall, O. M. (2005). Use of methylphenidate in traumatic brain injury. *Annals of Pharmacotherapy, 39*, 1309–1313.

Siever, L. J. (2008). Neurobiology of aggression and violence. *American Journal of Psychiatry, 165*, 429–442.

Silberstein, S. D. (2009). Preventive migraine treatment. *Neurologic Clinics, 27*, 429–443.

Smith, E. G., Sondergard, L., Lopez, A. G., Anderson, P. K., & Kessing, L. V. (2009). Association between consistent purchase of anticonvulsants or lithium and suicide risk: A longitudinal cohort study from Denmark, 1995–2001. *Journal of Affective Disorders, 117*, 162–167.

Snell, D. L., Surgenor, L. J., Hay-Smith, E. J., & Siegert, R. J. (2009). A systematic review of psychological treatments for mild traumatic brain injury: An update on the evidence. *Journal of Clinical and Experimental Neuropsychology, 31*, 20–38.

Spinella, M., Yang, B., & Lester, D. (2004a). Prefrontal system dysfunction and credit card debt. *International Journal of Neuroscience, 114*, 1323–1332.

Spinella, M., Yang, B., & Lester, D. (2004b). Prefrontal system dysfunction and credit card debt. *International Journal of Neuroscience, 117*, 301–313.

Stanford, M. S., Helfritz, L. E., Conklin, S. M., Villemarte-Pittman, N. R., Greve, K. W., Adams, D., & Houston, R. J. (2005). A comparison of anticonvulsants in the treatment of impulsive aggression. *Experimental and Clinical Psychopharmacology, 13*, 72–77.

Sztajnkrycer, M. D. (2002). Valproic acid toxicity: Overview and management. *Journal of Toxicology and Clinical Toxicology, 40*, 789–801.

Tomson, T., & Battino, D. (2009). Pregnancy and epilepsy: What should we tell our patients? *Journal of Neurology, 256*, 856–862.

Tucker, G. J., Price, T. R. P., Johnson, V. B., & McAllister, T. (1986). Phenomenology of temporal lobe dysfunction: A link to atypical psychosis—A series of cases. *Journal of Nervous and Mental Disease, 174*, 348–356.

Verrotti, A., la Torre, R., Trotta, D., Mohn, A., & Chiarelli, F. (2009). Valproate-induced insulin resistance and obesity in children. *Hormone Research, 71*, 125–131.

Vigo, D. V., & Baldessarini, R. J. (2009). Anticonvulsants in the treatment of major depressive disorder: An overview. *Harvard Review of Psychiatry, 17*, 231–241.

Wagner, K. D., Redden, L., Kowatch, R. A., Wilens, T. E., Segal, S., Chang, K., . . . Saltarelli, M. (2009). A double-blind, randomized, placebo-controlled trial of divalproex extended-release in the treatment of bipolar disorder in children and adolescents. *Journal of the Academy of Child and Adolescent Psychiatry, 48*, 519–532.

Wang, J. T., Shiu, G. K., Ong-Chen, T., Viswanathan, C. T., & Skelly, J. P. (1993). Effects of humidity and temperature on in vitro dissolution of carbamazepine tablets. *Journal of Pharmacological Science, 82,* 1002–1005.

Willmott, C., & Ponsford, J. (2009). Efficacy of methylphenidate in the rehabilitation of attention following traumatic brain injury: A randomized, crossover, double-blind, placebo controlled inpatient trial. *Journal of Neurology, Neurosurgery, and Psychiatry, 80,* 552–557.

Wilimowska J., Florek, E., & Peikoszewski, W. (2006). Disposition of valproic acid in self-poisoned adults. *Basic Clinical Pharmacology and Toxicology, 99,* 22–26.

Yerevanian, B. I., Koek, R. J., & Mintz, J. (2007). Bipolar pharmacotherapy and suicidal behavior. Part I: lithium, divalproex, and carbamazepine. *Journal of Affective Disorders, 103,* 5–11.

8

Blast Trauma: An Ominous "New" Risk Factor for MIND?

It was just like the Jolly Green Giant picked me up and shook me. I felt like a big "shaken baby."

—Anonymous war-fighter
(personal communication to R. J. Roberts)

Introduction

In previous chapters, we have focused almost exclusively on mild TBI due to blunt-force trauma. To review, this is the type of head trauma in which mechanical energy is applied directly to the skull (i.e., closed head trauma) or in which the skull is impelled at a significant rate of speed into a stationary object (e.g., telephone pole during a motor vehicle accident, concrete patio during a fall from a ladder). Blunt-force trauma represents the most common form of energy transfer to brain tissue, and most cases of MIND in civilian life likely are to be caused by this type of brain injury. However, other forms of excessive energy transfer to the brain deserve consideration in addition to blunt-force, mechanical trauma.

Blast-Induced Neuro-Trauma (BINT)

The major focus of this chapter is on what has been called "blast-induced neuro-trauma" (BINT) or explosive blast neuro-trauma (Ling, Bandak, Armonda, Grant, & Ecklund, 2009; Cernak & Noble-Hauesselein, 2010). Although large explosions likely have occurred in all wars fought since the invention of dynamite, the primary offensive weapon used by the enemy in the Global War on Terror (GWOT) has become the strategic use of the Improvised Explosive Device (IED) or Explosive Force Penetrator (EFP) to simultaneously kill or wound soldiers and disable their transport vehicles (Champion, Holcomb, & Young, 2009; Wolf, Bebarta, Bonnett, Pons, & Cantrill, 2009). It should be noted that higher energy explosives have been employed in IEDs and EFPs during the Global War on Terror than were used during World War I and World War II. Early in the wars in Iraq and Afghanistan, a typical IED consisted of 1–3 howitzer shells wired together with some C4 explosive or gasoline, a home-made bomb that is hidden along a roadside and remotely detonated by cell phones or electronic devices when American vehicles and troops are present. (In this chapter, the word "concussion" refers to a blast-concussion due to exploding ordnance rather than to a concussion of the brain. Although it is likely that blast-concussions do produce what neurologists and sports medicine physicians term "concussive brain injuries," in order to avoid confusion we have chosen to use the phrase "blast-concussion" TBI to refer to the mechanism of trauma rather than to describe the subsequent, disruptive effects upon brain function.) As greater proficiency has been achieved by our enemies in the later years of operations OIF and OEF, larger and more highly focused, roadside bombs have become more capable of penetrating protective armor on military vehicles and, thus, more deadly.

Instances of TBI due to blast-concussion have been labeled by the media as the signature injury of the OIF/OEF campaigns; however, such a description may be regarded as somewhat offensive by some veterans and their loved ones. It is clear that severe blast-concussion injury (i.e., from a large blast that occurs at close range) can be lethal to the brain and other organ systems. What is less clear at the present time is the extent to which soldiers who suffer brief loss of consciousness or who are merely dazed for some minutes experience persistent brain damage or dysfunction (Forsten et al., 2008). As the reader might imagine, given the long-standing and intense debate over mTBI due to blunt-force injury, opinions vary widely among clinicians and researchers on issues raised by possible blast-induced neurotrauma. With considerable under-statement, Dr. Deborah Warden, former chief neurologist at Walter Read Medical Center, concluded, "The vulnerability of the human brain to primary blast injury is controversial and an area of active research" (Taber, Warden, and Hurley, 2006).

When one logs on to YouTube on the Internet, types "IED Blasts," and then watches the numerous video postings (many of which are the work of the enemy) of American vehicles being hit, common sense dictates that blast-wave concussions would appear to be capable of producing brain injury in soldiers both outside and inside the targeted vehicles. Experts agree that being in immediate proximity to a *major* blast causes death due to brain damage and other forms of internal injury (Glasser, 2005). However, experts in good faith appear to be divided as to whether concussion-blasts can produce *bona fide* brain injuries when soldiers and Marines briefly lose consciousness or are simply stunned for short periods of time. (A few of the postings on YouTube have amazingly been shot by military personnel inside of vehicles while they are in the process of having their vehicles hit with IEDs. Such videos tend to corroborate the histories given by military veterans in similar circumstances who report to their care providers at military hospitals and DVA medical centers that, after recovering their senses and getting oriented, they continued to function, after a fashion, even though they felt dazed, suffered from acute hearing impairment, or experienced persistent headache.)

While employed primarily as a pediatric nephrologist (i.e., a physician specializing in kidney function in children), Ronald Glasser, M.D., has made an entire second career out of chronicling the nature of physical and emotional injuries suffered by American servicemen in the major wars our country has fought. In his 2005 book, *Wounded: from Vietnam to Iraq*, Dr. Glasser documented that major IED blasts generate unbelievably fast and extreme blast pressures at close range (Stewart, 2009). Glasser's numerous conversations with military physicians and surgeons have convinced him that the forces generated by IED blasts—even at a distance—can produce so-called mild TBI. His reasoning for drawing this conclusion is that the brain is like firm custard or jelly, but *jelly with differing densities*. Thus, when set in motion by a blast wave, tissues of differing densities will inevitably move at differing speed, presumably shearing and stretching axonal connections between neurons. More than one military surgeon reportedly stated to Dr. Glasser that they would prefer to suffer a missile wound through the head because the adverse effects of the injury would be limited largely to the track of the bullet or shrapnel, rather than diffusely distributed throughout the brain. Put another way, it is possible that the deleterious effects of a blast-wave exposure can have both global and focal components, whereas brain damage produced by an uncomplicated bullet wound to the brain itself is usually more focal should the war-fighter survive.

In his book, Glasser noted that:

> . . . soldiers walking away from blasts have later discovered that they suffer from memory loss, short-attention spans, muddled reasoning, headaches, confusion, anxiety, depression and irritability. . . . Army neurologists fear that subtle but real and related psychological problems are simply being missed in those troopers exposed to blasts but not visibly injured enough to enter the [in-country] medical evaluation chain. A 2005 medical paper on casualties resulting from blasts cautioned that with these injuries few are spared the blast effects of a car or roadside bomb. Indeed, the blast injuries to the brain should be expected in any soldier exposed to these explo-

sions, regardless of the distance from the blast center. It is the newest legacy of the newest American war . . . and a legacy that is growing each month. (p. 82)

At the level of the individual warrior, *USA Today* reporter Gregg Zoroya related the story of Marine Lance Corporal Gene Landrus who was injured in a May 2006, roadside bomb attack near Abu Ghraib, Iraq. Like many other combatants, Landrus apparently did not recognize that the memory loss, dizziness, nausea, and headaches he suffered likely were signs of brain injury. Nor, reportedly, did the Army medics who examined him. According to Zoroya (2007):

> Landrus was riding in an open-backed, armored Humvee when the roadside bomb detonated. It was his second exposure to a blast. An explosion a month earlier had "rung our bells a little bit, but no one was knocked unconscious." In the attack, Landrus and three other Marines blacked out for several seconds. After Landrus regained consciousness, "everything looked like it was going in slow motion," he recalled. . . .
>
> "I still can't remember what I did the day before or stuff that I did earlier in the day," he said. He carries a Palm Pilot or a pad of paper to write down orders, numbers or dates, so he can remember them later. The headaches have never gone away.
>
> Landrus will never fully recover, said Jessica Martinez, his lead therapist at Scripps [Memorial Hospital]. "This is basically like an invisible injury," she says. "He looks like a normal guy . . . But if you spend any amount of time with him . . . you would be able to notice that something's really happened. (p. 3)

Although some of Landrus's symptoms are consistent with the chronic symptoms of PPCS, his intermittent, abrupt memory lapses for events earlier in the day also are clearly consistent with the presence of MIND, as described in the present book. It appears as if this patient may have both episodic and chronic components to his memory deficits.

Ongoing Controversy Regarding Blast Exposures As a Cause of Brain Injury

In May 2006, Walter Reed Army Medical Center neurologist Deborah Warden and two colleagues published a review article titled, "Blast–Related Traumatic Brain Injury: What Is Known?" The answer they cautiously and correctly concluded was essentially, *not much*. They noted three potential major mechanisms of brain injury following nonfatal concussion blasts. First, there are rapid changes in atmospheric pressure following explosions, with the initial wave of pressure referred to as blast "over-pressure," followed by the subsequent development of a relative vacuum called blast "under-pressure." In their words, "Organs and tissues of different densities [e.g., white matter, gray matter, and cerebrospinal fluid] are accelerated at different rates, resulting in displacement, stretching and shearing forces" (p. 142). The second possible mechanism of injury they termed ballistic trauma, one that results from " . . . objects put in motion by the blast impacting a person." This notion is essentially similar to the notion of blunt-force trauma used in this article and includes shrapnel that hits a soldier's head or helmet (but does not penetrate the vault of the skull) and flying debris from the collapse of surrounding structures. Tertiary blast trauma occurs when an individual is blown out of a vehicle or up against a structure of some sort (e.g., impacting the metal body of a tanker truck by the explosive wind following a blast). This also is essentially a form of blunt-force trauma, conceptually similar to striking one's head on the windshield, steering wheel, or door frame during a motor vehicle accident. Thus, it seems clear that many patients with concussion-blast head trauma often sustain some degree of blunt-force trauma as well within the same blast episode. In addition to the three major causes of brain injury following blast, miscellaneous or quaternary blast injuries include all other types of injuries caused by explosions, such as burns, crush injuries, toxic inhalations, and medical misadventures. Additional details on the potential mechanisms from blast-concussion can be found in Forsten et al. (2008), Cernak and Noble-Haeusslein (2010), and Roberts (2008).

Several additional points deserve comment. First, unlike cerebrovascular accidents (or strokes), which tend to produce similar neurological deficits in patients based upon the portion of the brain that is affected adversely, no two episodes of so-called mild TBI due to blast-concussion are likely to generate highly similar clinical outcomes. For example, the driver of a Humvee who hypothetically is adjacent to a spot where an IED is detonated from 10 feet away may well experience a different long-term clinical outcome than the passenger next to him in the front seat, or the partially exposed gunner who hits his head on the turret, or a Marine outside the vehicle who has his helmet knocked off by the blast wave and then hits his head on the pavement. Furthermore, a charge that is detonated 10 feet adjacent to the driver of a Humvee is likely to have somewhat different clinical effects than an identical charge that is set off directly underneath the driver as he passes over it (John Meyers, Psy.D., personal communication, November 22, 2009).

Second, many combat veterans have been exposed to multiple IED blasts much like some professional football players have been exposed to multiple instances of blunt-force sports-concussions on the football field (Omalu et al., 2006). Although no exact dose-response curve can be established between number of instances of blunt-force mild TBI and the severity of clinical outcome in the individual case, most research studies using group statistics generally have demonstrated that multiple instances of blunt-force mild TBI are more likely to produce lasting cognitive and behavioral deficits than a single instance of blunt-force trauma. Put another way, it seems highly likely that more severe and more frequent IED blast exposures should produce more serious and long-lasting clinical problems, all other factors being equal. Future studies with experimental helmets with pressure sensors that are being tested in the field may provide needed data to address the effects of a single blast exposure versus multiple blast exposures. In the meantime, we agree with Cernak and Noble-Haeusslein (2010) that the pathophysiology of disrupted brain function following blast exposure is likely to be complex.

Finally, it is likely that many military personnel exposed to IED blasts also will have experienced separate instances of blunt-force head trauma in military or civilian life due mainly to motor vehicle accidents, falls, or previous sports concussions. Furthermore, when one is faced repeatedly with the prospect of being blown-up, shot, or kidnapped by the enemy, the development of clinically significant Post-Traumatic Stress Disorder (PTSD) is highly likely, and some experts believe that prolonged exposure to chronic and severe stress also may produce or promote damage or persistent dysfunction to the brain (e.g., Bremner, 2002). Throw in the possibilities of unknown toxic exposures, chronic dysentery and diarrhea, possible heatstroke, the undocumented effects of firing repeated mortar or howitzer rounds (Saljo, Arrhen, Bolouri, Mayogra, & Hamberger, 2008), and the effects of binge-drinking or illicit drug use as a recreational activity after discharge from the military and one begins to get a sense of the complexities which need to be considered when an individual combat veteran (or his family) insists that he or she is just not right after returning to civilian life from combat in southwest Asia.

As mentioned previously, not all experts are concerned equally about the longer term effects of blast-concussion. Hoge et al. (2008), for instance, suggested on the basis of survey data, that PTSD from combat was more likely to be associated with post-concussive symptoms than was reported history of mild TBI (i.e., the symptoms of PPCS were found to be more general and nonspecific rather than clearly diagnostic of mTBI). In fact, Hoge later went so far as to imply that the brain-trauma screening practices of the Department of Veterans Affairs (DVA) and Department of Defense (DoD) were a waste of clinical resources. Similarly, Wessely and his British colleagues (Jones, Fear, & Wessely, 2007) concluded that there was little evidence for the concept of shell-shock based upon a review of the literature from the two World Wars. Furthermore, based upon his own survey of military personnel from the United Kingdom, Wessely concluded:

> . . . PCS [post-concussive] symptoms are common and some are related to exposures such as blast injury. However, this association is not specific, and the same symptom complex is also related to numerous other risk factors and exposures. (p. 1641)

In a similar vein, an Australian psychiatrist, Wallace (2009), opined,

> Traumatic brain injury has been described as the "signature wound" of the current conflicts in Iraq and Afghanistan. While this term is highly debatable and probably unhelpful, clinicians need to know about this condition to provide the best management. (p. 218)

The conservative clinical advice of Australian neuropsychologist Richard Bryant, which already was quoted in Chapter 3 of this book, sternly cautions care providers against creating unduly pessimistic expectations among military combatants exposed to blast waves.

Fairly recent studies from investigators who have actually examined or tested blast-exposed patients (as opposed to using only survey methods) have provided some support for the proposition that blast-induced neuro-trauma is associated with longer term effects. Belanger and colleagues performed cognitive testing on matched groups of blast-exposed and blunt-force TBI patients and concluded that the neuro-cognitive test findings from both groups were highly similar. Colonel Heidi Terrio of the U.S. Army and her colleagues (Terrio et al., 2009) examined soldiers returning from Iraq and concluded:

> Following deployment to Iraq, a clinician-confirmed TBI history was identified in 22% of soldiers. . . . Those with

TBI were significantly more likely to report postinjury and postdeployment somatic and/or neuropsychiatric symptoms than those without this injury history. (p. 14)

Two observations about the results of Terrio's study are especially noteworthy. The first is that the observed rate of 22% at-risk for mild TBI is extremely close to the conclusion of the RAND study (Tanielian & Jaycox, 2008), which was conducted independently. The second is that, according to reporter Gregg Zoroya, the Department of Defense markedly increased its estimate of the likely number of brain-injured military personnel around the same time that Terrio's study was published.

A recent study from Madigan Army Medical Center in Washington indicated that almost all soldiers who suffered a concussion attributed to blast-exposure suffered from headaches for the next few months (cited in Hurley, 2009). A second study performed by Ruff and colleagues at the Louis Stokes VA Medical Center in Cleveland found that mild TBI due to explosion was often associated with neuro-cognitive deficits and a defective sense of smell (a clinical sign often associated with prefrontal damage) in veteran patients referred for evaluation and treatment of persistent headaches (Ruff, Ruff, & Wang, 2008). Finally, a small-scale neuro-imaging study using MRI with diffusion tensor imaging (a recent technical development that enhances the likelihood of finding structural brain lesions) showed that blast exposure was associated was associated with a pepper-spray pattern of small abnormalities in subcortical structures in white matter. Colonel Michael S. Jaffe of the U.S. Air Force, the primary investigator on this imaging study, was quoted as saying, "There is a different pattern we're seeing with a blast compared to the impact or acceleration-deceleration injuries, the type seen in motor vehicle accidents or athletic injuries" (quoted in Hurley, 2009).

Although comprehensive review of the relevant research from experimentation using animal models of blast exposure is beyond the scope of this book, note that such models have produced brain damage and dysfunction in at least two species, the rat and the pig (Saljo, Arrhen, Bolouri, Mayorga, & Hamberger, 2008; Saljo, Bolouri, Mayorga, Svensson, & Hamberger, 2010).

Thus, although there already has been considerable difference of opinion expressed regarding the possible longer term clinical significance of blast exposures, it seems possible, if not likely, that blast-concussions can produce damage or dysfunction in vulnerable brains (Cernak & Noble-Haeusslein, 2010; Ruff, Ruff, & Wang, 2008).

It is important for care providers to attempt to tease apart the relative effects of mild TBI and PTSD for a variety of reasons, including providing appropriate clinical treatment (Vaishnavi, Rao, & Fann, 2009) and assessing the disability status of blast-exposed veterans within the Department of Veterans Affairs. However, the most crucial reason is that both mild TBI and PTSD appear to make independent contributions to increased risk of suicide in such dually diagnosed patients (Gutierrez, Brenner, & Huggins, 2008; Jakupcak et al., 2009). Put another way, when both conditions are present, the risk of suicide likely is to be even greater than when just one of the two conditions is present.

In the next chapter, we continue to focus on blast-concussion and the possible role of symptoms of MIND in complicating recovery from mild TBI in combat veterans who have been exposed to blast waves.

References

Bremner, J. D. (2002). *Does stress damage the brain?* New York, NY: W.W. Norton.

Cernak, I., & Noble-Hauesselin, L. J. (2010). Traumatic brain injury: An overview of pathobiology with emphasis on military populations. *Journal of Cerebral Blood Flow and Metabolism, 30*, 255–266.

Champion, H. R., Holcomb, J. B., & Young, L. A. (2009). Injuries from explosions: Physics, biophysics, pathology, and required research focus. *Journal of Trauma, 66*, 1468–1477.

Forsten, R. D., Roberts, R. J., Stewart, C., Solomon, B. E., & Baggett, M. R. (2008). Assessing and treating veterans with traumatic brain injury. *Journal of Special Operations Medicine, 8,* 74–84.

Glasser, R. (2005). *Wounded: from Vietnam to Iraq.* New York, NY: Georges Brazillier.

Gutierrez, P. M., Brenner, L. A., & Huggins, J. A. (2008). A preliminary investigation of suicidality in psychiatrically hospitalized veterans with traumatic brain injury. *Archives of Suicide Research, 12,* 336–343.

Hoge, C. W., McGurk, D., Thomas, J. L., Cox, A. L., Engel, C. C., & Castro, C. A. (2008). Mild traumatic brain injury in U.S. Soldiers returning from Iraq. *New England Journal of Medicine, 358,* 453–463.

Hurley, D. (2009). Unique clinical, imaging findings seen among veterans with mild TBI. *Neurology Today, 9,* 18–20.

Jakupcak, M., Cook, J., Imel Z., Fontana, A., Rosenheck, R., & McFall, M. (2009). Posttraumatic stress disorder as a risk factor for suicidal ideation in Iraq and Afghanistan War veterans. *Journal of Traumatic Stress, 22,* 303–306.

Jones, E., Fear, N. T., & Wessely, S. (2007). Shell shock and mild traumatic brain injury: A historical review. *American Journal of Psychiatry, 164,* 1641–1645.

Ling, G., Bandak, F., Armonda, R., Grant, G., & Ecklund, J. (2009*).* Explosive blast neurotrauma. *Journal* of *Neurotrauma, 26,* 815–825.

Omalu, B. I., Dekosky. S. T., Hamilton, R. L., Minster, R. L., Kamboh, M. I., Shakir, A. M., & Wecht, C. H. (2006). Chronic traumatic encephalopathy in a national football league player: Part II. *Neurosurgery, 59,* 1086–1092.

Roberts, R. J. (2008, December–January). Impact on the brain. *Scientific American Mind,* 50–57.

Ruff, R. L., Ruff, S. S., & Wang, X. F. (2008). Headaches among Operation Iraqi Freedom/Operation Enduring Freedom veterans with mild traumatic brain injury associated with exposures to explosions. *Journal of Rehabilitation Research and Development, 45,* 941–952.

Saljo, A., Arrhen, F., Bolouri, H., Mayorga, M., & Hamberger, A. (2008). Neuropathology and pressure in the pig brain resulting from low-impulse noise exposure. *Journal of Neurotrauma*, *25*, 1397–1406.

Saljo, A., Bolouri, H., Mayorga, M., Svensson, B., & Hamberger, A. (2010). Low-level blast raises intracranial pressure and impairs cognitive function in rats: prophylaxis with processed cereal feed. *Journal of Neurotrauma*, *27*, 383–389.

Stewart, C. (2009). *Blast injuries: True weapons of mass destruction*. Tulsa, OK: Charles Stewart and Associates.

Taber, K. H., Warden, D. L., & Hurley, R. A. (2006). Blast-related traumatic brain injury: What is known? *Journal of Neuropsychiatry and Clinical Neuroscience*, *18*, 141–145.

Tanielian, T., & Jaycox, L. H. (2008). *The invisible wounds of war*. Santa Monica, CA: Rand Corporation.

Terrio, H., Brenner, L. A., Ivinas, B. J., Cho, J. M., Helmick, K., Scally, K., . . . Warden, D. (2009). Traumatic brain injury screening: preliminary findings in a U.S. Army Brigade Combat Team. *Journal of Head Trauma Rehabilitation*, *24*, 14–23.

Vaishnavi, S., Rao, V., & Fann, J. R. (2009). Neuropsychiatric problems after traumatic brain injury: Unraveling the silent epidemic. *Psychosomatics*, *50*, 198–205.

Wallace, D. (2009). Improvised explosive devices and traumatic brain injury: The military experience in Iraq and Afghanistan. *Australasian Psychiatry*, *17*, 218–224.

Wolf, S. J., Bebarta, V. S., Bonnett, C. J., Pons, P. T., & Cantrill, S. V. (2009). Blast injuries. *Lancet*, *374*, 405–415.

Zoroya, G. (2007, November 22). Marine didn't recognize signs of brain injury. *USA Today*, 3.

9

Blast Trauma II: Symptomatic Treatment in the Short-Run?

Okie (2006) refers to TBIs as the signature wound of this war. She reports that blasts are the most common form of soldier injuries, and, at the large Walter Reed Army Hospital, it has been found that 60% of those with blast injuries suffer from TBI. . . . This translates into thousands of lives affected now, with more to be affected as the war continues. And since soldiers have families, the ripple effect of TBIs through our nation will be monumental, and perhaps nation changing, as we cope to provide medical care and other types of support.

—Norman Keltner & Brandi Cooke (2007, p.223)

The Quest for Practical Knowledge About Blast-Exposure

The U.S. Congress has appropriated millions of dollars devoted to accelerating research on mild TBI, in general, and the effects of blast-concussion, in particular. Similarly, American veterans' organizations have called for more research in these areas. In the professional and scientific literature, almost all reviewers of the putative effects of nonlethal blast exposures on brain function conclude with calls for additional studies on this topic, one which is crucial to retired military veterans, active-duty fighters, and their families. Entire issues of scholarly journals, such as the *Journal of Neurotrauma* (June, 2009), have been devoted to articles regarding the development and refinement of scientific models of blast-concussion mTBI. The words of the guest editors of that issue of the *Journal of Neurotrauma* are fairly typical of the current zeitgeist. In an introductory article titled "A Critical Problem Begging for New Insight and New Therapies" (Kochanek, Bauman, Long, Dixon, & Jenkins, 2009), the authors wrote:

> As a consequence of the Iraq war, blast injury has reached a new level of importance due to the high numbers of these types of injuries seen in our warfighters, and includes a wide spectrum of them ranging from mild to severe. The pathophysiology of blast-induced TBI remains poorly understood, and is complicated by many factors such as repetitive exposure and superimposed polytrauma. . . . We must link the field, the bedside, and the bench, if those of us in the neurotrauma research community are going to discover the answers to the many questions that remain in this field, and to help develop new therapies to treat this condition. (p. 813)

Indeed, the U.S. government has been so eager to develop creative solutions that 300 million dollars have been allocated for alternative treatments, such as acupuncture and holistic medicine, to provide symptomatic relief for afflicted combat veterans.

If We Learn More About the Effects of Blasts, Then We'll Be More Able to Treat Those Effects More Adequately

The assumption underlying the development of animal research models of blast exposure and *structural* neuro-imaging studies of blast-exposed veterans (Warden, French et al., 2009) is that once researchers know what (if any) *structural* damage there is to the brain, then that information is likely to lead to improved treatment in a straightforward fashion. However, clinical science does not necessarily advance in such an orderly fashion (cf., Heath & Heath, 2007). In the words of neuroscientist Scott Small, "Knowing the mechanism is nice, but ultimately it's about curing the disease" (quoted by Halpern, 2007, p. 225).

Thus far, more research attention appears to have been paid to evaluating brain *structure* as opposed to brain *function*. Various aspects of brain *function* generally are measured by such diverse methods as electroencephalography (EEG or brain-wave recordings), neuropsychological testing, and *functional* neuro-imaging procedures such as Positron Emission Tomography or Single Photon Emission Computerized Tomography (PET and SPECT scans, respectively), which may be more likely to document brain dysfunction. The first published case study that used SPECT to study a multisymptomatic, blast-exposed veteran demonstrated clear abnormalities in the anterior regions of the brain (Harch et al, 2009). More recently, Peskind and colleagues (Peskind et al., 2010) used PET scan technology to compared the metabolic *function* of the brains of 12 Iraq war veterans with PPCS symptoms following one or more blast exposures to that of 12 matched control subjects. They concluded the following:

> Compared to controls, veterans with mTBI (with or without PTSD) exhibited subtle impairments in verbal fluency cognitive processing speed, attention, and working memory, similar to those reported in the literature for patients with cerebellar lesions. These FDG-PET imaging findings suggest that regional brain hypometabolism may constitute

a neurobiological substrate for chronic PCS in Iraq combat veterans with repetitive blast-trauma. Given the potential public health implications of these findings, further investigation of brain function in these veterans appears warranted.

Although these early studies using *functional* imaging techniques (as opposed to *structural* pictures of the brain) do not confirm whether or not some blast-exposed patients develop MIND (as suggested in Roberts, 2008), the results suggest that *functional* neuro-imaging techniques (or the combination of functional and structural neuro-imaging techniques—see Huang et al., 2009) are more likely to demonstrate changes in brain activity following blast exposure than are structural neuro-imaging techniques.

So What Do We Do Now?

Currently, blast-exposed combat veterans already fill the clinics of both Department of Veterans Affairs and Department of Defense medical centers. As reservists and National Guard members continue to depart Asia, and as more American soldiers and Marines leave the military, blast-exposed patients increasingly will visit the offices of civilian practitioners as well. In the absence of a clear consensus or clinical guidelines as to how to evaluate and treat blast-exposed patients, care providers are faced with "doing their best" to provide symptomatic treatment based upon what we already know.

One of the methodologically soundest and most persuasive studies of relevance to the longer term effects of blast-concussion in combat was published by Trudeau and his associates in 1998 —three years *prior* to the global war on terror (Trudeau et al., 1998). For reasons that are not apparent to the authors of this book, this study has been seldom cited during the debate over the possible effects of blast-concussion. Trudeau compared performances on several measures from a group of 27 veteran patients with histories and PTSD and mild TBI due to blast exposure with those from a group of 16 veteran patients with PTSD but no histories of blast-exposure mild TBI. One of the measures reflecting the electrical activity of the brain was called quantitative EEG (abbreviated qEEG). Based upon a type of statistical analysis called discriminant function, quantitative EEG data correctly identified 88% of the blast-positive subjects and 75% of the blast-negative subjects (i.e., those who suffered from PTSD without a history of mTBI due to blast-concussion). In addition, the blast-positive patients performed significantly worse on a measure of sustained attention (the Test of Variables of Attention). Furthermore, members of the blast-positive group rated themselves as having greater attentional difficulties in everyday life relative to the blast-negative control subjects. Most of the subjects studied were Vietnam veterans, as well as some Korean War veterans. The results remained essentially the same, even when the potential effects of alcohol use were taken into account statistically.

Although the authors of the study described their research as "exploratory," several points deserve comment:

1. It seems likely that there may be longer term problems with brain *function* following blast-concussion in combat.

2. Some portion of such putative dysfunction likely is electrical in nature, reflecting underlying changes in electrophysiological activity that are not prominent on standard EEG (i.e., no clear evidence of epilepsy or seizures) but can be detected by a more fine-grained computer-analysis (quantitative EEG).

3. Both objectively (when sustained attention was tested) and subjectively (when questionnaires on attention were completed), veteran patients with blast-positive histories demonstrated evidence of poorer attentional functioning years after the acute blast.

4. Studies using quantitative EEG would appear to be worth performing in the current generation of OIF/OEF combat veterans, who have been exposed to blast waves; however, thus far none have been published.

Unfortunately, Trudeau's research group, to our knowledge, has not produced any replication or further extension of their provocative study from 1998.

At the present time, the authors of this book do not possess any systematic experimental data to suggest that some of the symptoms reported by blast-exposed combat veterans are due to MIND. However, because of the widespread nature of the problem and the call for new insight and new therapies (Kochanek et al., 2009), we feel that it is appropriate to inquire, in a clearly speculative fashion, whether *some*, but not all, blast-exposed veterans referred for neuropsychological evaluation might endorse experiencing multiple intermittent symptoms of MIND, similar to those endorsed by blunt-force trauma patients with MIND (Roberts, 2008).

In addition to obtaining histories of blunt-force head trauma and blast exposure, VA Poly-Trauma clinics typically employ a 22-item checklist to screen combat veterans for Post-Concussive Symptoms (Schwab et al., 2007). The content of this symptom inventory is presented in Table 9–1. These items are essentially post-concussive symptoms (as opposed to the episodic symptoms of MIND).Veterans are asked to rate how much each symptom has "disturbed you" on a 5-point scale, ranging from No Disturbance/Rarely (0) to Very Severe Disturbance (4). (Please note that this is a subjective judgment of *severity*, not a *frequency rating*, as required by the Iowa Interview.) Based upon the presence of persistent post-concussive symptoms and other interview information, it then is decided whether a blast-exposed veteran should be referred for neuropsychological assessment or other diagnostic measures.

It is our impression that most neuropsychologists seldom interview specifically for *intermittent symptoms* with an instrument such as the Iowa Interview (Roberts, 1999), even when

Table 9-1. Post-Concussive Symptom Items from the Neurobehavioral Symptom Inventory (NSI) for Screening Troops Returning from Deployment in Afghanistan and Iraq

- Feeling dizzy
- Loss of balance
- Poor coordination, clumsy
- Headaches
- Nausea
- Vision problems, blurring, trouble seeing
- Sensitivity to light
- Hearing difficulty
- Sensitivity to noise
- Numbness or tingling in part of my body
- Change in taste and/or smell
- Increased or decreased appetite
- Poor concentration, cannot pay attention, easily distracted
- Forgetfulness, cannot remember things
- Difficulty making decisions
- Slowed thinking, difficult getting organized, cannot finish things
- Fatigue, loss of energy, cannot finish things
- Difficulty falling or staying asleep
- Feeling anxious or tense
- Feeling depressed or sad
- Easily annoyed/irritability
- Poor frustration tolerance, feeling easily overwhelmed by things

From: Schwab, K. A., Ivins, B., Cramer, G., Johnson, W., Sluss-Tiller, M., Lux, W., & Warden, D. (2007). Screening for traumatic brain injury in troops returning from deployment in Afghanistan and Iraq: Initial investigation of the usefulness of a short screening tool for traumatic brain injury. *Journal of Head Trauma Rehabilitation, 22,* 377–389.

screening has established that a particular patient has persistent post-concussive symptoms. This state of affairs is understandable since few neuropsychologists have been taught or trained to pay attention to such symptoms; however, this situation is unfortunate because, as neuropsychiatrist Fred Ovsiew (2008) has pointed out, many neuropsychiatric patients (including those with traumatic brain injuries) experience spell-like phenomena with abrupt onset and offset—the sorts of events that we have been referring to as *intermittent symptoms* in this book. In Ovsiew's words:

> Many "spells" or "attacks" occur in neuropsychiatric patients, and taking the history of a paroxysmal event has certain requirements regardless of the nature of the event. . . . For any attack disorder, how frequent and how stereotyped the events are should be determined. Rapidity of onset and cessation, disturbance of consciousness or of language; occurrence of autochthonus sensations, ideas, and emotions and of lateralized motor or cognitive dysfunctions; purposeless movements and coordination of actions; memory for the spell; and duration of the recovery period should be ascertained. (p. 139)

Ovsiew goes on to list the Iowa Interview (Roberts, 1999) as one of the instruments that is useful for assessing such intermittent symptoms.

There likely are several reasons why many neuropsychologists and other types of care providers do not pursue intensively interviewing for intermittent symptoms following head trauma. As mentioned previously, formal academic training often does not emphasize the assessment of neurobehavioral symptoms that come and go with the same degree of emphasis that is paid to the assessment of chronic symptoms that are more-or-less always present. Also, until perhaps the past decade, patients with traumatic brain injury were thought to be poor case material for studying how the normal brain actually works, when compared with more discrete forms of neurologic disease such as stroke patients or those with neurosurgical resections. Additionally, some clinicians, particularly those with active forensic practices and those who believe they have been deceived by patients in the past, seem to express considerable skepticism with regard to the usefulness of verbal report data from patients with multiple complaints (Axelrod, 2006; Jones, 2006). Finally, with no formal definition of the diagnosis of MIND in either the psychiatric or neurologic diagnostic nomenclature, many practitioners are skeptical that a single patient can experience so many intermittent symptoms without having a major psychosis, somatization disorder, malingering/exaggeration, or compensation neurosis. The intermittent symptoms that such patients do describe spontaneously tend to be dismissed or discounted as "medically unexplained physical symptoms" (Jones & Wessely, 2005).

The first author of this book recently has published a case study (Roberts, 2008) of a blast-exposed, military veteran with significant symptoms of MIND. This patient responded positively to clinical treatment with an anticonvulsant mood-stabilizer (valproic acid or Divalproex). That case, as well as the case history to be presented here, demonstrates that some patients with symptoms of PPCS following blast exposure may respond favorably to combined treatment with an anticonvulsant mood stabilizer and an antidepressant.

Case Study. Paul experienced three blast exposures during his tour in Iraq; these were reported to be at distances of roughly 50 yards away, 15 feet away, and at close range. The latter blast resulted in shrapnel injuries to his body (but not his head). When he returned stateside, an initial neuropsychological evaluation conducted by a civilian neuropsychologist attributed Paul's "mild cognitive problems" to "anxiety and depression" associated with "readjustment" to civilian life. As the months passed by, Paul's problems with irritable outbursts at work and home worsened, leading to a referral to a VA neuropsychologist for a second opinion.

When seen for the second neuropsychological assessment, the veteran complained at length during an open-ended interview about his excessive irritability, unpredictable cognitive lapses (which he colorfully termed "brain-farts") and severe headaches. He reported that he had quit or been fired from six jobs since returning from Iraq and felt his current marital situation was tenuous. He had become so irritable at home that his spouse reportedly had even sanctioned his use of alcohol in off-hours because it seemed to dull his irritability and help him fall asleep, even though she generally was opposed to such use.

Re-analysis of the test data from the first neuropsychological exam and additional neurobehavioral testing provided evidence of clinically significant attentional dysfunction (i.e., poor immediate or working memory), psychomotor slowing, inconsistent performances on short-term memory and learning tasks, and right partial anosmia with reported hypogeusia. In addition, the patient's performance on an auditory, divided-attention task, dichotic listening, was *grossly* defective (below the 1st percentile), despite normal hearing on pure-tone audiometry. (Past research with mild TBI due to blunt-force trauma has demonstrated that defective dichotic listening performance likely is associated with electrophysiological dysfunction.)

Somewhat uncharacteristically for most blast-exposed combat veterans in whom structural neuro-imaging evaluations typically are read as being unremarkable, Paul's MRI was found to have small white-matter lesions of "uncertain etiology." Unfortunately, Paul was not referred for *functional* neuro-imaging studies such as PET or SPECT scans.

On a commonly used screening device for PCS, the Rivermead Post-Concussive Scale, Paul obtained an extremely high score (47/64), with multiple items endorsed as "severe" problems. This elevated score was consistent with the presence of PPCS.

On a semistructured interview of intermittent or episodic symptoms, the Iowa Interview, Paul obtained an abnormal score of 72 (i.e., well above the 95th percentile cutoff score of 50 in the pathological direction). With regard to individual intermittent symptoms, he endorsed the following intermittent symptoms with *clinically significant frequency* (i.e., at or above the 90th percentile of the normal control distribution for each particular item):

- Gustatory illusions

- Olfactory illusions

- The illusion of movement in peripheral vision, episodic tingling in uninjured body parts

- Episodic tinnitus

- Unexplained episodes of brief cephalic pain

- Episodic dysarthria

- Word-finding lapses

- Brief memory gaps

- Unrecalled conversations with other people

- Brief staring spells witnessed by others

- Unexplained, profuse nocturnal sweating

- Severe nightmares

- Unprovoked, ego-dystonic mood swings (i.e., *not* triggered by PTSD stimuli)

The results of the second interview and neuropsychological exam were noted to be generally consistent with the effects of a mild TBI due to blast-concussion. (It is important to remember that so-called mild TBI refers only to the acute response of the brain to the traumatic event and *not* to the severity of longer term outcome for the patient.)

During a separate interview with a combat-trauma specialist, Paul *also* was diagnosed with combat-related PTSD and secondary depression. He subsequently was treated by his psychiatrist with valproic acid (Divalproex) for his temper, rapid mood swings, and cognitive lapses and was later prescribed doxepin (Sinequan) for his frequent, persistent headaches by a consulting neurologist. With this combination of an anticonvulsant mood stabilizer and an antidepressant medication, Paul gradually became less irritable at home, experienced fewer headaches, and eventually reached the point where he could significantly reduce his alcohol intake. He and his spouse then were able to engage meaningfully in marital therapy sessions that did not degenerate into angry verbal outbursts on his part. He maintained his job as a baker and did well while attending a special culinary school.

Paul ultimately received an 80% service-connected pension for a combination of PTSD, residual effects of traumatic brain disease, and tinnitus. Coping with the stresses of civilian life remained effortful, but temper control and subjective well-being all improved following the strategically timed combination of initial pharmacotherapy and later behavioral interventions. Note that none of this patient's health-care providers regarded Paul as manifesting a conventional form of epilepsy.

When considered together, the favorable results from the previous case study (Roberts, 2008) and the case study presented in this chapter suggest that the combination of a mood stabilizer with anticonvulsant properties and an antidepressant medication may provide symptomatic relief for some military veterans who endorse significant symptoms of MIND in the post-acute period following blast exposure.

To be prudent and even-handed, it must be acknowledged that we currently lack systematic data on the endorsement of episodic symptoms on the Iowa Interview following blast exposure. Furthermore, although there has been at least one double-blind, randomized controlled study of treating depressed mood following blunt-force TBI with Sertraline, an SSRI antidepressant (Ashman et al., 2009), the authors are unaware of any such study for either an antidepressant or a mood stabilizer with anticonvulsant properties for mood problems following blast exposure. The only empirical evidence we could find regarding the combination of an antidepressant and mood stabilizer with anticonvulsant properties was a study by Pasquini and his colleagues (Pasquini et al., 2007). These investigators found that unipolar psychiatric patients with significant irritability responded favorably to open trials of such a combination of medications. Unfortunately, there was no information in their article about possible histories of head trauma prior to treatment.

In summary, it seems likely that some post-concussive symptoms following blast exposure may remit with the passage of time for most patients (Terrio et al., 2009). However, individual patients with mild TBI may continue to report persistent dysfunction following blast exposure (e.g., Thompson, Scott, & Dubinsky, 2008). Interviewing systematically for intermittent symptoms in cases of PPCS is one option open to the evaluating clinician (Roberts, 2008). In such cases, when there also is comorbid PTSD from combat and the prescribing clinician and patient agree to attempting an empirical trial of treatment with valproic acid (Divalproex), it seems likely that significant improvement is most likely to reflect a reduction in symptoms of MIND because the best evidence suggests that valproic acid has little or no positive impact on uncomplicated PTSD (Davis et al., 2008; Hamner et al., 2009). It also is important to note that Packard (2000) has presented evidence that divalproex can be an effective agent in preventing persistent post-traumatic headaches. Furthermore, both divalproex and carbamazepine have been used effectively to treat cases when impulsive (or explosive) anger is a prominent presenting component (Lux, 2007). One argument for treating symptoms of MIND prior to those of PTSD is to explain to the skeptical patient that the brain dysfunction associated with MIND is like an amplifier in a home entertainment system, an entity that "turns up the volume" on the symptoms of PTSD and thereby amplifies human suffering. That is why the symptoms of MIND may need to be dealt with prior to intensive treatment for PTSD.

In the next chapter, we discuss behavioral strategies and tips for coping with residual life problems associated with mild TBI and MIND, after the symptoms of MIND have been treated optimally with medications.

References

Ashman, T. A., Cantor, J. B., Gordon, W. A., Spielman, L., Flanagan, S., Ginsberg, A., Engmann J., . . . Greenwald, B. (2009). A randomized controlled trial of sertraline for the treatment of depression in persons with traumatic brain injury. *Archives of Physical Medicine and Rehabilitation, 90,* 733–740.

Axelrod, B. N. (2006). Interpreting symptoms in military personnel after combat. *Lancet, 367,* 1709–1710.

Davis, L. L., Davidson, J. R., Ward, L. C., Bartolucci, A., Bowden, C. L., & Petty, F. (2008). Divalproex in the treatment of posttraumatic stress disorder: A randomized, double-blind, placebo-controlled trial in a veteran population. *Journal of Clinical Psychopharmacology, 28,* 84–88.

Halpern, S. (2007). *Can't remember what I forgot: The good news from the front lines of memory research.* New York, NY: Harmony.

Hamner, M. B., Faldowski, R. A., Robert, S., Ulmer, H. G., Horner, M. D., & Lorberbaum, J. P. (2009). A preliminary controlled trial of divalproex in posttraumatic stress disorder. *Annals of Clinical Psychiatry, 21,* 89–94.

Harch, P. G., Fogarty, E. F., Staab, P. K., & Van Meter, K. (2009). Low pressure hyperbaric oxygen therapy and SPECT brain imaging in the treatment of blast-induced chronic traumatic brain injury (post-concussion syndrome) and post traumatic stress disorder: A case report. *Cases Journal, 9,* 6538.

Heath, C., & Heath, D. (2007). *Made to stick: why some ideas die and others survive.* New York, NY: Random House.

Huang, M., Theilman, R. J., Robb, A., Angeles, A., Nichols, S., Drake, A., . . . Lee, R. R. (2009). Integrating imaging approach with MEG and DTI to detect mild traumatic brain injury in military and civilian patients. *Journal of Neurotrauma,* April 22, Epub ahead of publication.

Jones, E., & Wessely, S. (2005). War syndromes: The impact on medically unexplained symptoms. *Medical History, 49,* 55–78.

Jones, R. (2006). Interpreting symptoms in military personnel after combat. *Lancet, 368,* 838.

Keltner, N. L., & Cooke, B. B. (2007). Biological perspectives: Traumatic brain injury-war related. *Perspectives in Psychiatric Care, 43*(4), 223-226.

Kochanek, P. M., Bauman, R. A., Long, J. B., Dixon, C. R., & Jenkins, L. W. (2009). A critical problem begging for new insight and new therapies. *Journal of Neurotrauma, 26,* 813–814.

Lux, W. E. (2007). A neuropsychiatric perspective on traumatic brain injury. *Journal of Rehabilitation Research and Development, 44*, 951–962.

Ovsiew, F. (2008). Bedside neuropsychiatry: Eliciting the clinical phenomena of neuropsychiatric illness. In S. C. Yudofsky & R. E. Hales (Eds.), *The American Psychiatric Publishing textbook of neuropsychiatry and behavioral neurosciences* (5th ed., pp. 137–187). Washington DC, American Psychiatric Publishing.

Packard, R. C. (2000). Treatment of chronic daily headache with divalproex sodium. *Headache, 40*, 736–739.

Pasquini, M., Picardi, A., Speca, A., Orlandi, V., Tarsitani, L., Morosini, P., . . . Biondi, M. (2007). Combining an SSRI with an anticonvulsant in depressed patients with dysphoric mood: An open study. *Clinical Practice of Epidemiology in Mental Health, 8*, 3–10.

Peskind, E. R., Petrie, E. C., Ross, D. J., Pagulayan, K., McCraw, K., Hoff, D. . . . Minoshima, S.(2010). Cerebrocerebellar hypometabolism associated with repetitive blast exposure mild traumatic brain injury in 12 Iraq war veterans with persistent post-concussive symptoms. *Neuroimage, 10*, E-pub prior to publication.

Roberts, R. J. (1999). Epilepsy Spectrum Disorder in the context of mild traumatic brain injury. In N. R. Varney & R. J. Roberts (Eds.), *The evaluation and treatment of mild traumatic brain injury* (pp. 409–447). Mahwah, NJ: Lawrence Erlbaum.

Roberts, R. J. (2008, December–January). Impact on the brain. *Scientific American Mind*, 50–57.

Schwab, K. A., Ivins, B., Cramer, G., Johnson, W., Sluss-Tiller, M., Lux, W., & Warden, D. (2007). Screening for traumatic brain injury in troops returning from deployment in Afghanistan and Iraq: Initial investigation of the usefulness of a short screening tool for traumatic brain injury. *Journal of Head Trauma Rehabilitation, 22*, 377–389.

Terrio, H., Brenner, L. A., Ivins, B. J., Cho, J. M., Helmick, K., Schwab, K. . . . Warren, D. (2009). Traumatic brain injury screening: Preliminary findings in a US Army Brigade Combat Team. *Journal of Head Trauma Rehabilitation, 24*, 14–23.

Thompson, J. M., Scott, K. C., & Dubinsky, L. (2008). Battlefield brain: Unexplained symptoms and blast-related mild traumatic brain injury. *Canadian Family Physician*, *54*, 1549–1551.

Trudeau, D. L., Anderson, J., Hansen, L. M., Shagalov, D. N., Schmoller, J., & Nugent, S. (1998). Findings of mild traumatic brain injury in combat veterans with PTSD and a history of blast concussion. *Journal of Neuropsychiatry and Clinical Neuroscience*, *10*, 308–313.

Warden, D. L., French, L. M., Shupenko, L., Fargus, J., Riedy, G., Erickson, M. E., . . . Moore, D. F. (2009). Case report of a soldier with primary blast brain injury. *Neuroimage*, *47*(Suppl.), T152–T153.

10

Using Effective Coping Behaviors

*Although only a minority of individuals who have sustained
a mild traumatic brain injury develop persisting . . .
symptoms, the impact on their psychological well-being
and everyday functioning can be considerable. The importance
of developing cost-effective interventions which are acceptable
to the patient cannot, therefore, be underestimated.*
                                                    —Elizabeth Allen (2007, p.181)

In our experience, effective treatment of MIND with medication(s) does not mean that all intermittent symptoms completely disappear. Nor does it mean that patients treated successfully do not need to take extra effort to do things that used to come more automatically. The purpose of this chapter is to provide coping tips for dealing with problems that remain and for avoiding common pitfalls. The tips are numbered for the reader's convenience, but not necessarily in order of importance for the individual patient. Practicing and using *some* of these tips may not be necessary for *some* individuals. However, it cannot hurt to have reviewed them all at least once by reading the entire chapter. If you are a patient who lives with a significant other, it also may be useful to have that person read this chapter and then consider his or her input.

1. **Try to live a very consistent life from day to day.** The major difference between a single-celled animal (like an amoeba) and a human being is that the amoeba is completely dependent on the content of the fluid around it for meeting its basic biological needs. Unlike the amoeba, human beings carry our own "sea water" around inside us. Much of the physiological activity in our bodies is directed at maintaining the chemical content of the fluids in our bodies within fairly narrow limits, a biological process called *homeostasis*. Anything that adversely affects the chemical content of our bodily fluids (e.g., blood, cerebrospinal fluid) carries with it a risk for producing or exacerbating problems with brain function. Therefore, patients with MIND should *try* to eat regular, balanced meals, avoid excessive exercise in extreme heat, drink sufficient fluids, restrict alcohol intake, and maintain a regular sleep cycle. These recommendations are said more easily than done in our fast-paced, postmodern world.

   Furthermore, an injured brain has less tolerance for wide variations in basic biological functions when compared to the uninjured brain, even when the effects of the injury have been treated optimally with medication. It becomes more important to live a relatively consistent life guided by the principle, "Everything in moderation."

2. **Compliance, compliance, compliance.** If the motto for success in real estate is "location, location, location," then the mantra for successful treatment of MIND should be "compliance, compliance, compliance." For medical purposes, the word "compliance" refers to taking medications (and following other instructions) as prescribed. As children, most of our early experiences were with medications such as ibuprofen or acetaminophen—ones

in which you take the medicine and about 20–30 minutes later you feel better. That is, pain is lessened, fever is reduced, or some other desired effect becomes noticeable within a fairly short amount of time. In contrast, the effectiveness of most mood-stabilizing medications (and most antidepressant medications) depends upon gradually reaching, and then maintaining, a stable target level of the medication in the bloodstream. That is why the full effects of some medications are not apparent until a patient has been taking a certain dosage for several weeks (i.e., an adequate trial of treatment). That is also why it is important to take medications in the correct dose at the times they are scheduled. If a patient with MIND is having difficulty remembering to take medication as prescribed, then it is often helpful to temporarily enlist a family member or friend to assist in reminding the patient when to do so. Put another way, until the taking of medications becomes habitual for the patient, the other person should be placed in charge of ensuring medication compliance. Also, a variety of watches with beeping reminder functions and pill boxes with timers are now available to help patients remember to take their medications on time.

3. **Plan for exceptional circumstances.** When you pack to go out of town, or even for an overnight stay, remember to pack your prescription medications first, so you do not find yourself in unfamiliar territory without your medications. Should this occur, it is sometimes possible to negotiate with a local pharmacy or emergency room to obtain a partial prescription so that you do not experience discontinuation syndrome (i.e., similar to what used to be called withdrawal effects). If you know you are going to be gone from home for an extended period of time (e.g., semester abroad, extended vacation), then it is important to make arrangements with your insurance company and your pharmacist to receive enough

medication in advance to maintain compliance through the period of time you will be away from home.

4. **Consider keeping one day's worth of medication locked in the glove compartment of your vehicle.** Mornings can prove to be a very hectic time for busy families and an easy time to overlook taking medication. If you have one day's worth of each type of medication with you, then you won't get stuck at work or college without your morning dosage, should you have forgotten to take it at home before you left. It is important to keep such spare medications locked up so that young children do not find them by accident. Also, if you are in the habit of sleeping at more than one location on various nights, then try to keep a small medicine bottle or medicine tray with you each day.

5. **It is virtually always better to use a week-long medication planner or tray.** This way, medications can be put in the tray once per week, and you always know where you can find them. Also, when you take your medications directly out of their bottles, you may forget or become uncertain whether you took them earlier in the day. When pills are all laid out for the week, it becomes much easier to determine whether or not you have already taken a set of medications for that day. Once again, whatever system you use for storing your medications, be sure to keep them out of the reach of children.

6. **Under extremely hot weather conditions, blood levels of medication may sometimes fall.** With hot summer weather or excessively warm working conditions when large amount of fluids are consumed, blood levels of certain medications may fall, especially if you work under very hot conditions (e.g., the way roofers, construction workers, or factory workers may do). If the blood level of mood-stabilizing medication falls for any

reason, you may be prone to experiencing more frequent or severe intermittent symptoms. If this happens,
you need to contact your prescribing physician for
advice.

7. **Sometimes medications levels may drop with diarrhea.**
   If you have an illness, such as stomach flu, with diarrhea
   or frequent bowel movements, lower levels of certain
   medications may be absorbed due to the medication
   being cleared from your system much more quickly.
   Sometimes intermittent symptoms can break through
   or become more frequent. Again, if you think this might
   be happening, check with your prescribing physician.

8. **If you frequently have to search for your personal
   belongings, then there needs to be "a place for everything and everything in its place."** Part of absent-
   mindedness is simply getting home or getting to the
   workplace and putting one's belongings down any-
   where that's handy. Certain patients with mild TBI end
   up spending a great deal of time searching for personal
   possessions such as keys, watches, rings, wallets, purses,
   glasses, cell phones, and even computers or personal
   daily assistants (PDAs). The individual who is prone to
   memory lapses needs to develop a system for setting
   down and then locating key personal belongings. One
   way to accomplish this is to designate a particular box
   or container to hold all such items when you are at
   home. You need to place your frequently used belongings in that container *as soon as you come in the door—*
   before you get distracted by anything else. Everything
   you use on a regular basis should go right into the container—and nowhere else. That way, it becomes a habit
   you can rely on. Similarly, if you know you will be
   receiving or dealing with a good deal of paperwork
   from one source (e.g., Social Security, Department of
   Veterans Affairs, Internal Revenue Service, Medicare,
   Workman's Compensation), it is good to get in the habit

of storing that paperwork with all the paperwork from the same source in the same designated file or organizer right after you open it and read it. Important deadlines can be missed due to lost or misplaced paperwork, and such delays can mean a loss of benefits or delays in obtaining benefits to which you are entitled.

9. **If you use an electronic device, such as a Blackberry, Palm Pilot, PDA, laptop computer, or programmable cell phone as a memory aid, make sure that all crucial information is backed up or printed out in hard copy somewhere.** Many types of electronic devices can be used successfully to cope with memory problems, particularly for individuals who enjoy new technologies. However, you do not want to be stranded if your electronic device gets broken, misplaced, stolen, or is otherwise unavailable. Having to start over from scratch can be very time consuming. Also, if your memory-assisting device runs on batteries, make sure that you have a spare set fully charged and ready to go.

10. **If you do not like to use electronic devices as reminders, consider taking a small, pocket-sized notebook and a pen with you at all times so you can write down instructions and things you need to do** *as soon as you are told.* That way, you are less likely to forget job assignments or important appointments. When you get back home, transfer all future appointments or time-related information to *just one calendar* or daily planner (as opposed to multiple calendars for different types of events). Try to check the calendar (or have someone remind you to check the calendar) at least twice a day. Always put your calendar, planner, or electronic memory aid in the same place.

11. **Try to remove clutter from your life.** If a piece of junk mail comes, throw it away after you or your significant other has made the determination that it has no future

value. After you finish reading a newspaper, set it in a box to be recycled rather than leaving it on the sofa. Other than *financial* records, *medical* records, records from *military service,* and *legal* papers, chances are good that, if you haven't used something in nine months, you may not need it. As your living space becomes less cluttered, then it probably will be easier to find things when you do misplace them. Try to sort and group similar papers together, such as financial records with financial records, pay stubs with pay stubs, communications from Social Security with other communications from Social Security—as mentioned previously. *Avoid hoarding useless or excessive personal possessions, such as old magazines or newspapers.*

12. **If you have to learn new material for your job or your education, avoid waiting until the last minute.** Try to read or study when your mind is rested or at its most efficient. Doing chores or watching mindless TV can come later when there is less need to concentrate. Do mental work when your concentration is at its best. Don't try to cram at the last minute. A quiet place that is free from distractions (e.g., a den, an empty classroom, or a secluded desk in a library) can help you stay focused. If you are not under time pressure and have multiple assignments or projects to tackle, *start with the most difficult one first*—that way, everything else that follows will be easier or more pleasant. A number of briefer, spaced learning sessions (e.g., multiple half-hour time blocks) separated by rest or relaxation periods are likely to prove more beneficial than a single session of massed practice lasting several hours. Don't be afraid to ask others for help.

13. **You needn't feel ashamed of your remaining symptoms or problems, but don't be afraid to apologize either.** When you experience a memory lapse (such as forgetting someone's name or getting lost in the middle of

a sentence during a conversation), try not to feel ashamed. After all, you did not ask to have this happen; in most instances, your intermittent symptoms occur because you had some sort of accident and hit your head. However, do not be afraid to make a brief apology or explanation to others ("I'm sorry, what was I just saying?" or "I have difficulty with people's names. Could you please tell me you name again?"). Some individuals apparently have learned to equate making an apology with showing weakness to others. If this is the case, you may need to sit down with a counselor or some other type of care provider to actually practice when and how to make minor apologies, so it begins to feel more natural and familiar. No one is perfect, and everyone makes mistakes sometimes.

14. **Pay active attention to learning people's names.** If learning the names of new people has become difficult for you, try to say the new person's name aloud as soon as possible (e.g., "Nice to meet you, Ms. Reynolds.). Then try to rehearse the new person's name two to three times silently in your mind so it is more likely to stick. Try to use the person's name once or twice in conversation to rehearse it aloud. When you are in a meeting or class with more than 4 or 5 new people, have a clean sheet of paper ready so you can diagram the room and write down everyone's name as they introduce themselves. Then you do not have to rely on your short-term memory when you need to address someone in the room.

15. **If you are attending school or enrolled in some sort of formal educational program, before you begin classes, check with the Office of Student Services or Student Disability Services to determine whether you are entitled to any reasonable accommodations during your education.** Depending upon your circumstances, you may be eligible for more time to take a test, tutoring

services, note-taking services, recording teachers' lectures, or other types of assistance based upon remaining cognitive problems associated with your head injury. However, the college or institution that you are attending may request that you sign a Release of Information form for past medical records. The office of disability services also may require that you undergo some formal testing to demonstrate what specific accommodations are needed under the scope of the Americans with Disabilities Act.

16. **If you suffer from intermittent rage outbursts, try to remove yourself from your family (or the immediate social environment), if possible, when you sense that a rage outburst may be coming on.** Although memory lapses and headaches tend to be the most distressing MIND symptoms for patients, family members often are most distressed by temper outbursts that are excessive or appear to come out of nowhere. Sometimes an abrupt loss of temper simply occurs without warning; however, at other times, patients can sense that they are at increased risk for "losing it." In the latter situation, try to remove yourself from stressful circumstances, get off by yourself, and try to calm down or distract yourself. Unless your personal safety or that of your loved ones is immediately at stake, it is usually best if you can refrain from acting in a hostile, aggressive fashion, even if that action consists of only screaming at someone. And once again, apologizing for startling other people or hurting their feelings is entirely appropriate if you do lose your temper in front of others in a public situation. If you find yourself losing control repeatedly, you should consult your physician or care provider for additional recommendations. If you know that certain situations have the potential to be anger-provoking (e.g., dropping children off with an ex-spouse following weekend visitation, shopping in a large and crowded

mall), try to make plans to avoid those potential anger-triggers if they are indeed avoidable.

17. **Strongly consider abstaining entirely from drinking alcohol (or using illicit drugs).** Alcohol is a central nervous system depressant, and it temporarily raises seizure threshold while it is in the bloodstream. After the alcohol is metabolized and excreted from your system, however, seizure threshold is lowered, making it more likely that your brain will become electrically unstable. (With severe drinking problems, alcohol-withdrawal seizures tend to occur when a *severe* alcohol abuser *stops* drinking regularly.) Returning to the analogy of the amoeba and the "sea water," any steps a MIND patient can take to keep the chemical content of their body as stable as possible probably will pay off in terms of the patient having fewer symptoms and life problems. On the other hand, cycles of consuming alcohol and then not consuming alcohol are likely to interfere with both the positive effects of medication and the electrical stability of one's brain.

18. **If you have quit reading out of frustration over forgetting what you have just read, you may need to ease your way back into it.** One way gradually to improve your reading retention is to go to your public library and find a book that interests you and that the library also has on cassette tape or CD. That way you can follow along visually with the text while you listen to the narrator read the same words. Just make sure that the tape or CD version of the book has not been edited or abridged (so that the text from the page will be identical to the narration). Eventually, after you are used to following the printed text again, you gradually can try weaning yourself off the narrated version of the story for longer and longer periods of time. Some libraries are too small to have their own collections of books on tape or CD, but, when requested, most libraries will

order such materials from a larger library on an inter-library loan request.

19. **Avoid getting cocky or overconfident regarding your need for ongoing medication.** Sometimes when MIND patients have been treated effectively for an extended period of time, they have difficulty remembering how much worse life was prior to treatment with medication. Some patients may be tempted to "play doctor" and take themselves off of their medications without consulting their physician because it feels like they don't need them any longer. It is virtually *always* a mistake to attempt to manage one's own medications without contacting your physician. First, the reduction in medication may not be called for. Second, many medications that have direct effects upon the brain need to be tapered gradually, so that the patient does not experience discontinuation syndrome and symptoms of withdrawal. Third, the extent to which medication can be reduced or withdrawn without relapse and return of previous intermittent symptoms is currently unclear (Neppe & Kaplan, 1988). After a favorable treatment response has been established, it sometimes can be difficult to re-establish an equally favorable response even when the same medications at the same dosages are restarted by the treating physician.

20. **Avoid getting angry and throwing all your medicines away.** Even patients whose lives have been improved with treatment still get very angry, at times. Occasionally, patients threaten to throw their medications away or flush them down the toilet in protest or for some irrational reason (e.g., getting back at the government, a care provider, or a spouse). This impulsive course of action almost always ends up hurting the patient himself and distressing those around him. It is similar to the old phrase, "cutting off one's nose to spite one's face." Once again, before making any changes in your

medication regimen, give yourself time to calm down and check with your physician. Simply doing this can save everybody more distress. Furthermore, flushing pills down the toilet contributes to certain medications being found in public water supplies. If you do have to dispose of old medications that are no longer prescribed, check with your pharmacist about an environmentally friendly way of doing so.

21. **Try not to overtax yourself in a way that ends up disturbing your sleep pattern.** Some people need more rest following a head injury. Excessive fatigue and need for sleep are fairly common problems following even mild TBI. So, *guard your sleep.* Try to make decisions that do not end up putting your normal sleep pattern at risk, such as staying up late to study or partying all night. Similarly, driving a car all through the night to reach a distant destination sooner is *never* a good idea. Whenever possible, choose to work a typical daytime shift, rather than a night shift; working nights may pay slightly more money, but it can complicate or disrupt your sleep cycle. If you have been told by others that you have a serious snoring problem and that you stop breathing for brief periods of time at night, you should tell your physician, as these symptoms may reflect a sleep apnea syndrome. Similarly, if your sleep is disrupted at night by sudden jumping and twitching of your legs, you should also tell your physician, as these could be signs of restless legs syndrome. In either case, your physician may suggest an overnight sleep study at a nearby medical center.

22. **Try to focus on one task at a time.** Multitasking often results in fragmented or poorer task performances for individuals without a history of TBI. Case studies (e.g., Bootes & Chapparo, 2010) suggest that having to split one's focus of attention on more than one task may be even more difficult for individuals following persistent

mild TBI. Thus, structuring one's educational or vocational time to decrease interruptions and distractions (when possible) may facilitate task performance.

23. **Guard your head.** A single instance of mild TBI, like that sustained in 2009 by actress Natasha Richardson, is seldom fatal. However, a rare, clinical entity called Second Impact Syndrome (Bey & Ostick, 2009), in which an individual (often an athlete) sustains a second impact within a week of a prior impact, can be fatal. The second impact can result in diffuse cerebral swelling, brain herniation, and death—sometimes within just a few minutes. Even when less dramatic, the outcome of an additional head injury can exacerbate markedly the effects of a previous head injury. Therefore, patients who have experienced residual difficulties following an episode of persistent PPCS, persistent mild TBI, or complicated concussion should take special care to avoid sustaining future head trauma. Even seemingly innocuous activities such as sledding, cycling, water- or snow-skiing, horseback riding, or getting hit in the head with a hardball while playing baseball can aggravate the effects of previous head injury. If one is unwilling to forego such activities, then care should be taken to wear an appropriate helmet. (For example, if you care enough about biking to buy an expensive mountain bike, there is little sense in buying the cheapest helmet possible.) Although this is only our opinion, if you have sustained clinically significant head trauma, you should strongly consider avoiding motorcycling altogether because of its risk for head injury. The same is true for riding snowmobiles and four-wheelers at high speeds, at night, or over terrain that is unfamiliar or uneven. When operating other types of motor vehicles, always use seatbelts, ensure your airbags are connected and functioning properly, and drive at speeds appropriate for hazardous road conditions. While driving, actively

concentrate on operating your vehicle and avoid distracting yourself with answering cell phones, eating, applying make-up, shaving, or multitasking in other ways. Never text-message or Tweet while driving.

24. **Remember:** *guard your head! And the heads of those you love!*

References

Allen, E. A. (2007). Interventions for postconcussion syndrome. *Trauma, 9*, 181–187.

Bey, T., & Ostick, B. (2009). Second impact syndrome. *Western Journal of Emergency Medicine, 10*, 6–10.

Bootes, K., & Chapparo, C. (2010). Difficulties with multitasking on return to work after TBI: A critical case study. *Work, 36*, 207–216.

Neppe, V. M., & Kaplan, C. (1988). Short-term treatment of atypical spells with carbamazepine. *Clinical Neuropharmacology, 11*, 287–289.

11

Assessing Intermittent Symptoms After Pediatric Mild TBI

Because symptoms caused by mild TBI last less than half an hour, . . . the study of mild TBI is often neglected resulting in a significant knowledge gap for this wide-spread problem. In this work, we studied functional (electrophysiological) alterations of the neonatal/juvenile hippocampus after experimental mild TBI . . . the age of the tissue at injury was found to be an important factor affecting posttraumatic deficits in electrophysiological function, indicating a relationship between developmental status and vulnerability to mild injury. Our findings suggest that mild pediatric TBI could result in functional deficits that are more serious than currently appreciated.

— Zhe Yu & Barclay Morrison III (2010, p. 499)

Auras are insubstantial [sic], they are reports of a subjective experience given by one person to be understood by another. To elicit them from a patient who is reluctant to talk about them requires time and talent, and a belief in their importance.

— David C. Taylor & Moira Lochery (1987, p.677)

Introduction

It now is accepted generally that a subset of children and adolescents will not recover spontaneously from concussion or mild traumatic brain injury (Taylor et al., 2010). In research studies, the percentage of pediatric patients who will continue to have persistent post-concussive symptoms typically ranges from 15 to 30% of patients (e.g., Ponsford et al., 1999). Such a wide variation likely is due to sample selection (e.g., including as research subjects consecutive referrals to an emergency trauma center who have experienced *only one* concussion versus referrals to specialists in physical medicine and rehabilitation who generally have not recovered from the *most recent* concussion, regardless of past history of brain injury or neurologic illness) and type of research study (e.g., epidemiologic study that examines thousands of records to establish population prevalence versus clinical study of the cognitive outcome of sports concussion in a high school football team). In some studies, the proportion of children who do not recover fully has been even higher than 30% (e.g., Agrawal, Gowda, Bal, Pant, & Mahapatra, 2005; Roberts, M. A., 1999) because a high-risk sample (e.g., those who have experienced multiple concussions) was selected as the clinical group of interest.

Many of the previous research studies in this area (e.g., Max et al., 2004) have *excluded* children as subjects if they had sustained more than one mild TBI or had a history of neurologic illness. However, recent research (e.g., Guskiewicz et al., 2003; Theriault, DeBeaumont, Tremblay, Lassonde, & Jolicoeur, 2010) studying concussion outcomes (in collegiate contact sports such as football) has demonstrated convincingly that those young adult athletes who sustained more than one concussion require a longer time to recover, may experience highly persistent post-concussive symptoms, and necessarily require a longer time before return to play—if they are able to return to play at all. Satz and others (Fay et al., 2010; Satz, 1993) have proposed the concept of "brain reserve," which postulates that central nervous system injury and illness reduces brain reserve, and an individual with reduced brain reserve has less capacity to recover from subsequent trauma or neurologic illness. Research studies that select only those subjects who have experienced one concussive episode may not tell us much about the children in the "miserable minority" who have experienced persistent post-concussive symptoms because they are such a small proportion of their overall study group. For this reason, it is our contention that these high-risk patients are precisely the ones we should select to study if we are going to better predict which children are at risk for persistent problems and why. With such information, the potential for the development of more effective treatment methods would be greater.

In some cases, pediatric concussion goes undetected. Clinically, it is often necessary to ask basically the same question (i.e., Has your child/Have you experienced a concussion or multiple concussions?) in a number of different ways. In one clinical case treated by the chapter authors, the patient's aunt was told of the head trauma by the patient's sister. The sister was a witness to her brother being thrown from an all-terrain vehicle while riding on rough ground. Although the patient had a helmet on, it was not properly fastened, and it flew off during the accident. The patient was dazed and led into the house by his sister. After lying down for about an hour, the patient got up and appeared to be fine. This incident was not mentioned to the boy's father when he came to pick up his children. Over the next several months, a new onset of difficulties with attention and memory were noticed by teachers. The probable concussion was never even considered as a cause, because it was unknown to parents and teachers.

In the chapter authors' clinical experience, post-concussion symptoms also may be misinterpreted, as in the case of a teenager who was viewed by high school teachers as being unmotivated. Post-concussion symptoms also may be misattributed to other causes or diagnoses, such as Attention-Deficit/Hyperactivity Disorder. Adolescent patients may not mention that they hit their head or got "dinged" in a sports practice because they wanted to play in the next game; they just shook it off and tried to tough it out; or they simply did not recognize the symptoms or significance of experiencing a concussion (McCrea, Hammeke, Olsen, Leo, & Guskiewicz, 2004). Children and teens are more likely to experience concussion over the summer months when playing or participating in unsupervised sports activities. These events may not be witnessed by an adult and, thus, are likely not to be reported to school personnel in the fall. For those pediatric patients who are eventually referred to a neuropsychologist for evaluation, successful resolution of symptoms will depend on the examiner's familiarity with common developmental disorders and the ability to rule these diagnoses in or out as contributing factors.

If a child does not have an abrupt onset of significant symptoms (e.g., severe headache that does not respond to over-the-counter analgesics, severe memory problems in a well-behaved, high achieving, high school student), the concussion may be forgotten or dismissed as having been a minor event without consequence. In children, the onset and worsening of symptoms may be more gradual, as is exemplified in one case study published by the first author (Roberts, Manshadi, Bushnell, & Hines, 1995). In this case, intermittent symptoms following a whiplash injury developed gradually and became worse over a period of many months. Long-term treatment with counseling and antidepressant medication initially proved unsuccessful. Functional neuro-imaging (Positron Emission Tomography, PET) eventually documented significant bilateral hypo-metabolism in the mesial temporal lobes.

Concussions in children and adolescents most often occur during play or participation in sports. A blow to the head (e.g., helmet-to-helmet contact in football) or a fall (e.g., collision during basketball with one or both athletes falling and hitting their heads on the floor) may result in the acute symptoms of concussion, including brief loss of consciousness, period of post-traumatic amnesia, temporary visual loss or double vision, headache, nausea and vomiting, and balance difficulties. Sideline assessment by an athletic trainer or team physician may be available to athletes in team sports. Computerized sideline assessments such as ImPACT (e.g., Schatz, Pardini, Lovell, Collins, & Podell, 2006) may be administered. Alternatively, the trainer or physician can assess for acute neurologic symptoms, check orientation (in an age appropriate fashion), and ask questions about recent game activity (e.g., who scored the last goal, what quarter are we in). Inaccurate response to any of the questions asked, any abnormalities in any portion of the exam conducted, or any acute symptoms (e.g., nausea, balance problems) should result in the athlete being taken out of play until all symptoms resolve. Under the guidance of the child's physician, the patient may be monitored at home for 24 hours, as long as symptoms do not become worse, and they do resolve over that period of time. Some pediatric patients may be taken to the local emergency treatment center for additional evaluation.

Initial medical evaluation of the concussion often begins after the child has reached the emergency treatment center. A detailed history of the acute event, as well as a history of prior head trauma or neurologic illness should be obtained. Often, computerized tomographic scan (CT scan), X-rays, and neurologic exam also are completed. Abnormality on any of these measures is likely to result in hospital admission. Neurosurgical consultation and intervention also may be necessary. In most cases, the patient is discharged after a brief hospital stay (i.e., often one to two days), unless there are neurologic or orthopedic complications. Since the majority of children and adolescents recover from concussion, after they are discharged, no further medical follow-up may be scheduled.

In the present authors' hospital setting, the majority of hospitalized children are referred to the pediatric neuropsychologist for consultation. Initial evaluation is conducted, including age-appropriate extended testing of orientation and amnesia (e.g., Children's Orientation and Amnesia Test, Ewing-Cobbs, Levin, Fletcher, Miner, & Eisenberg, 1990), and testing of basic language functions, such as confrontation naming, verbal fluency, sentence repetition, and comprehension (e.g., Token Test) from the Multilingual Aphasia Exam (Benton, & Hamsher, 1989). Neuropsychological deficits identified can be addressed with educational accommodations in the early return to school (Roberts, M. A.,

1999). More extensive outpatient neuropsychological evaluation is available for those children who have not fully recovered in the first few months after the head trauma.

Among those children or teens who have not completely recovered from concussion, many may go months or years before successful identification, treatment, or resolution of their symptoms. If the concussion(s) have been identified at the time of symptom onset, a post-concussion symptom checklist or interview may have been administered. However, post-concussion symptom checklists or interviews often query for the trait-like behaviors or symptoms of developmental psychopathology. During this extended period of evaluation time and having seen multiple clinicians, the child may have received multiple psychiatric diagnoses (American Psychiatric Association, 1994) including Attention-Deficit Hyperactivity Disorder, Intermittent Explosive Disorder, Depressive Disorder, and Cognitive Disorder–Not Otherwise Specified. As presented in chapters 1 through 5, the persistent post-concussive symptom complaints are episodic rather than chronic. The acronym MIND (Multi-symptomatic Intermittent Neurobehavioral Disorder) was selected to call attention to the variable nature of symptom complaints following mild head trauma. The complicated issues surrounding effective treatment of pediatric patients with the persistent post-concussive symptoms of MIND are addressed in detail in the next chapter. However, treatment with stimulants or atypical antipsychotics is largely unsuccessful in treating the symptoms of MIND. In our experience, most young children are not prescribed SSRI antidepresssants for treatment of mood difficulties. However, some teens may derive benefit from such treatment when prescribed in conjunction with the preferred treatment for MIND patients—a mood stabilizer with anticonvulsant properties (e.g., carbamazepine or valproic acid).

For research purposes, the way in which we study assessment of pediatric mild TBI and the questions we ask in each study have a major impact on the outcomes we find. The following study method is common. Researchers seek to establish the frequency of psychiatric diagnoses (i.e., based on the current edition of the *Diagnostic and Statistical Manual of Psychiatric Disorders*) in three matched (i.e., often matched on the basis of time since injury, socioeconomic status, age at injury, gender, etc.) groups of children (i.e., moderate to severe traumatic brain injury, mild traumatic brain injury, and orthopedic injury groups). Investigators using such a study design typically have found, not surprisingly, that compared to the mild TBI group and the orthopedic injury group, those subjects who sustained severe traumatic brain injuries are more likely to fit the diagnostic criteria for trait-like developmental psychopathology. The severely injured children also are more likely to demonstrate some *recovery of function* (e.g., basic daily self-cares, walking, toileting, dressing). For decades, this has been a guiding principle in pediatric brain injury research; that is, post-injury symptoms can be attributed *only* to the injury if they demonstrate a degree of recovery after the injury. This approach may be misguided, however, because it attempts to fit the post-concussive symptoms to an already established, developmental, psychiatric diagnosis.

A New Clinical Framework

Perhaps we should be studying this problem with a different frame of reference, one other than developmental psychopathology. In an exhaustive review of the neurophysiology of concussion, Shaw (2002) concluded that the most likely causative explanation of post-concussive symptoms was electrical misfiring, similar, but not identical, to a seizure disorder. Research by Cohen and colleagues (Cohen et al., 2007) supports Shaw's conclusion that failure to recover from mild TBI can disrupt neuronal synaptic circuits:

> . . . In the hippocampus, research now suggests that TBI regionally alters the delicate balance between excitatory and inhibitory neurotransmission in surviving neurons, disrupting the normal functioning of synaptic circuits. In another approach, a simplified model of neuronal stretch

injury *in vitro*, has been used to directly explore how injury impacts the physiology and cell biology in the absence of alterations in blood flow, blood brain barrier integrity, or oxygenation associated with in vivo models of brain injury. This chapter discusses how these two models alter excitatory and inhibitory synaptic transmission at the receptor, cellular, and circuit level. . . . (p. 143)

R. J. Roberts and colleagues (Roberts, R. J., et al., 1992) provided a compelling comparison and contrast of MIND-like symptoms and the symptoms of traditional partial complex seizures. In support of this framework, Agrawal, Gowda, and others (Agrawal et al., 2005; Gowda et al., 2006; Umile, Sandel, Alavi, Terry, & Plotkin, 2002) have proposed that pediatric post-concussive symptoms result from temporal lobe dysfunction. Using SPECT or PET imaging, Agrawal and colleagues (Agrawal et al., 2005; Gowda, et al., 2006) and M. A. Roberts and colleagues (Roberts, Bushnell, Manshadi, & Hines, 1996) reported hypo-perfusion or hypo-metabolism, respectively, in the temporal lobes in pediatric patients with persistent intermittent symptoms.

The book's second author has had clinical experience with pediatric mild TBI for more than two decades. Interviews with parents and teachers have documented that the children with intermittent symptoms are *not consistently* angry, aggressive, hallucinating, nor inattentive. In fact, it is often the very unpredictable, episodic nature of these symptoms that makes them so difficult to deal with at home and school. The emotional outbursts that occur are typically out of proportion to the provocation (and may occur without provocation at all) and are out of character for well-behaved children. The individual child is often very apologetic after an extreme temper outburst or convincingly may not recall even having had the outburst at all. Hallucinatory (or illusory) experiences reported by children are generally not threatening, violent, or disintegrative (as is the case with a child with developing schizophrenia); rather, they are perceived as irritating and confusing. It should be acknowledged that a number of teenagers with visual illusions after a concussion are often hesitant to admit to having such illusions for fear that the evaluating clinician may diagnose them as psychotic or "crazy." In addition, a number of post-concussive symptoms reported do not fit well with the accepted criteria for trait-like, developmental psychopathology. Parents have reported brief staring spells, abrupt cessation of some activity, and memory gaps for conversations about positive events (e.g., an upcoming shopping trip). Teachers have reported children exhibiting behaviors contradictory to traditional reinforcement paradigms (e.g., student being given his coat to put on and go home [i.e., escape from demands of school setting] while fatigued and staring after a temper outburst, and this student pointlessly aggresses against the teacher who brought him his coat). Factor analytic studies of post-concussion questionnaires (e.g., Ayr, Yeates, Taylor, & Browne, 2009) reveal that children's symptom complaints load on the dimensions of somatic, cognitive, and emotional, which are similar to the main dimensions identified on the Iowa Interview.

Interview Assessment of Pediatric MIND

Based on M. A. Roberts's clinical experiences, more than a hundred items were generated to comprise a questionnaire for parents and teachers to complete about their child or student with a history of brain injury. A study regarding the Pediatric Inventory of Neurobehavioral Symptoms (PINS) (Roberts, M. A., 1992) was first published with preliminary norms in 1997 (Roberts & Furuseth, 1997). The results of that study demonstrated that episodic symptoms were significantly more frequent in a group of children with brain injury than either the normative group or a group with diagnosed Attention-Deficit/Hyperactivity Disorder (but no history of head trauma). The PINS was revised, and redundant items were eliminated with the assistance of Dr. Jerome Sattler for publication in the fourth and fifth editions of his classic text on the cognitive and behavioral assessment of children (Sattler, 2002; Sattler, 2006). One of the five rationally derived dimensions of the PINS included 12 items (score range from 0 to

36) and was labeled episodic symptoms (Table 11–1). In a group of 237 elementary students from Midwestern communities (Roberts, Wright, & Roberts, 2006), the 90th percentile cutoff was a score of 7. Four of the episodic symptom items most frequently were reported in those pediatric patients with persistent post-concussive disorder: (1) new onset of anger outbursts out of character for the child and out of proportion to the situation; (2) staring spells with memory gaps for the period of the staring spells; (3) tinnitus and sensitivity to bilaterally noisy environments (e.g., school cafeteria); and (4) headaches or head pains that did not resolve with traditional over-the-counter analgesics. Using these four items as screening questions and obtaining negative responses to these questions, it is unlikely in the authors' clinical experience that the residual post-concussive symptoms fall in the subtype of MIND (Multiple Intermittent Neurobehavioral Dysfunction, see Chapter 1) as described in the present book.

A second method of assessing the episodic symptoms following pediatric concussion also was being tested during the same time period as the PINS. R. J. Roberts and colleagues had developed and published the Iowa Interview (Roberts, R. J., 1999), which has been described in earlier chapters and in Technical Appendix I. A questionnaire form of the Iowa Interview (administered under the general title of Behavior Symptom Questionnaire with a score in the range of 0 to 180) also was developed by R. J. Roberts to obtain normative data on the Iowa Interview items from large groups of individuals. Roberts, Wright, & Roberts (2006) presented the Behavior Symptom Questionnaire's (BSQ) findings regarding MIND-like symptoms' rates in pediatric normative and high-risk mild TBI groups. Data from this study revealed that intermittent symptoms as described by the BSQ were uncommon in the normative group (90th percentile was a score of 9 or greater; 95th percentile was a score of 17 or greater). Sixty-four percent of the high-risk mild TBI group scored at or above the 95th percentile.

When employing the BSQ modification of the Iowa Interview to assess a child's or adolescent's persistent symptom complaints following concussion, clinical experience suggests some

Table 11-1. Episodic (i.e., Intermittent) Symptom Items from the Pediatric Inventory of Neurobehavioral Symptoms (PINS)

Item Number	Item Content
2	Reacts to minor events as if they were catastrophes
5	Complains of headaches or sharp head pains
19	Complains of hearing ringing, buzzing, or tapping noises
24	Says or does things unexpectedly, out of the blue, that are unrelated to what is going on
25	Complains of food tasting or smelling bad or rotten when the food is not bad or rotten
30	Sometimes stares off, unaware of what's going on around him or her
31	Has temper tantrums for no real reason over things that usually are not a big deal
36	Complains of seeing things that other people cannot see
41	Sometimes seems confused, but the confusion lasts only a short time
46	Feels sad or cries for no reason; has no explanation for the sad feelings
49	Has quick and dramatic mood changes (extremely happy one minute, extremely sad the next)
51	Seems to forget having had conversations with people

Note. Each item is scored from 0 (almost never or not at all) to 3 (very often or very much). For norms, refer to: Roberts, M. A., & Furuseth, A. (1997). Eliciting parental report following pediatric traumatic brain injury: Preliminary findings on the Pediatric Inventory of Neurobehavioral Symptoms. *Archives of Clinical Neuropsychology, 12*, 449–457.

From: Roberts, M. A. (1992). The Pediatric Inventory of Neurobehavioral Symptoms (PINS). Iowa City: University of Iowa.

age-specific considerations. Some items on the Iowa Interview are recognized mainly by others in the child's environment. For example, a parent or teacher likely will be able to report with a reasonable degree of accuracy on the frequency of staring spells or the precursors (even if minor) to an anger outburst. The child is often unaware of the frequency of staring spells or may deny that they occur at all. Similarly, the child may not recall what made him so angry or what he did during the episode (e.g., throwing objects at someone, a teenager punching a hole in drywall). In contrast, only the child may be able to report on the internal subjective experience of intermittent tinnitus and its frequency. When interviewing children, the usual caveat about using understandable or age-appropriate vocabulary should be noted here. If asked about episodic tinnitus, the child likely will give you a puzzled look. However, asking the child whether they ever hear a ringing or buzzing noise out of nowhere (i.e., no one around them is making such a noise) is likely to result in a more valid response. Estimating frequency with elementary age children might be better understood if the interviewer asks how many times during each school week does this ringing or buzzing noise happen. Also, some items may require translation into children's experiences. An excellent example of this is the item about automatic driving from the Iowa Interview. It has been our experience that such automatic behaviors do occur in children, but they manifest as wandering out of the house without knowing where they are going, pointlessly walking in the hallways at school, or taking off on a bike or scooter in pouring rain with no clear destination in mind.

Risk Factors for Persistent Dysfunction

Identification of those children and adolescents who are most at risk for developing the MIND subtype of persistent post-concussive disorder would represent an important advancement for early diagnosis and treatment. If physicians in the emergency treatment center were better able to predict those children who will not recover fully, these children could be followed more closely and treated earlier in the development of symptoms, with the result of an improved quality of life for all children with mild TBI and a reduced financial burden on the health-care system.

As has been mentioned earlier in the book, a cascade of metabolic changes occurs during the acute period following concussion (Giza & Hovda, 2001). Biological markers have been studied, including the APOE-4 allele in genetics, which has been linked to risk for other neurologic illness such as Alzheimer's. Proteins in blood, such as S100B, also have been examined as they predict the risk for poor outcome following concussion. To date, however, none of these biological markers has demonstrated significant potential for identification of those children who will make up the miserable minority (Geyer, Ulrich, Gräfe, Stach, & Still, 2009; Moran et al., 2009; Piazza et al., 2007).

Functional neuroimaging procedures, such as Single Positron Emission Computed Tomography (SPECT) or Positron Emission Tomography (PET), measure the perfusion of oxygen in blood flow or metabolism of glucose, respectively, in selected brain regions. These two *functional* neuro-imaging methods have demonstrated promise as potential biomarkers of poor outcome. Agrawal and colleagues (Agrawal et al., 2005, Gowda et al., 2006) reported the results of acute (i.e., within 72 hours of injury) and longer term (i.e., at 3 months post-injury) SPECT scans with children. During the acute period, approximately one-half of the subjects who participated demonstrated abnormalities of oxygen perfusion, most often in the temporal lobes. These pediatric subjects then were split into two groups, the group with perfusion abnormalities on SPECT and the group without perfusion abnormalities on SPECT. The children were again evaluated at 3 months post-injury. The group with abnormal SPECT scans during the acute period following injury also demonstrated abnormal SPECT scans at three months, and, most importantly, also demonstrated persistent post-concussive symptoms. Of the group with normal SPECT scans during the acute period, none of these children demonstrated abnormalities on SPECT at 3 months post-injury. In addition, only one child in the normal SPECT group was reported to experience post-concussive symptoms at three months. Additional research is needed to replicate these findings at other medical centers. Thus, at the present time, utilizing SPECT scans in the emergency treatment center is not really viable as a clinical assessment tool. However, this method does hold promise as a biological predictor of poor outcome following mild TBI in children. Temporal lobe hypo-perfusion also may support an etiological explanation and suggest potential medical treatment strategies.

Some researchers have examined the relative risk of a number of factors, including the child's history of prior injury, gender, and age at injury; acute medical symptoms; and performance on neuropsychological testing (Dick, 2009; Yeates, & Taylor, 2005; Yeates et al., 2009). M. A. Roberts (2006) presented the results from a study of 120 children and adolescents who had sustained one or more instances of mild TBI. Approximately 50% had been referred clinically for neuropsychological evaluation, and the remaining 50% had served as research participants. Children whose acute medical complaints included vomiting, dizziness, nausea, vision problems (e.g., temporary loss of vision, double vision), unilateral weakness, or balance problems were twice as likely as those without these complaints to have persistent post-concussion symptoms of the MIND subtype. Those participants who reported a history of experiencing three or more concussions (including the index concussion) during childhood or adolescence were three times as likely to have persistent post-concussion symptoms when compared to those participants who experienced no previous or only one concussion prior to the index concussion (the most recent concussion of study). One of the more provocative findings from this research suggested a "temporal window of vulnerability" (i.e., a span of time during which a child is highly likely—in the present group, 90% likely—to experience persistent post-concussive symptoms, often soon after the second concussion) in children, as has been demonstrated in animal models of mild TBI (e.g., Longhi et al., 2005; Vagnozzi et al., 2008). Graphing the distribution of the time interval between the index injury and the one preceding it demonstrated a three-month window of vulnerability. That is, the child who experienced two concussions within a three-month time span was almost certain to experience persistent post-concussive symptoms of the MIND subtype. Those children for whom greater than three months had elapsed between concussions did not have this greatly increased risk of poor recovery. Replication of these results is needed to support or disconfirm this three-month window of vulnerability. It would, however, allow early identification of those children at greatest risk of developing the MIND subtype.

Neuropsychological Evaluation

Results from neuropsychological evaluations of children with persistent problems following mild TBI often reveal memory deficits, particularly verbal memory deficits (e.g., Levin et al., 2008; Levin et al., 2004; Ponsford et al., 1999). Age at injury may have an impact on memory testing results because adolescents are more likely to show memory difficulties than younger children. Also, preschoolers who have sustained a mild TBI may later show deficits in perceptual skills and learning to decode letter symbols with beginning reading instruction in kindergarten and first grade (Gronwall, Wrightson, & McGinn, 1997; Wrightson, McGinn, & Gronwall, 1995), or they may later demonstrate pragmatic language deficits (Gerrard-Morris et al., 2010). Deficient performance on the Dichotic Word Listening Test (Roberts, Springer, & Roberts, 1990) has been associated with persistent post-concussive symptoms of the MIND subtype (Roberts, M. A., et al., 1994; Roberts, Manshadi, Bushnell, & Hines, 1995; Roberts, Verduyn, Manshadi, & Hines, 1996). M. A. Roberts's clinical experience suggests that the Dichotic Word Listening Test may not be as predictive of persistent post-concussive MIND symptoms for the individual elementary age child. Furthermore, it is difficult to obtain reliable results on children younger than 7 years with this task (Roberts, M. A., et al., 1994). However, when scores on the Dichotic Word Listening Test are abnormal (i.e., the child's score in repeating words presented to either the left or right ear is below normative expectations) in the absence of a clear structural lesion, it is highly likely that the child also will endorse troublesome intermittent symptoms of the MIND subtype when the family and child are interviewed.

Although most standard neuropsychological test findings are unremarkable in pediatric mild TBI (e.g., cognitive level on standard intelligence testing), there have been some unique cases of specific learning difficulties that had an abrupt onset after experiencing two concussions within the projected three-month window of temporal vulnerability. In one instance, a high school sophomore fell from his bike while riding on a dirt path. He was not wearing a helmet and was reported to have hit the back left quadrant of the skull. Three weeks prior to this event, the young man had fallen while rollerblading (once again, without a helmet), striking the left parieto-occipital area. This young man had a history of being an A-student, active in extracurricular events, with supportive family and friends, and no changes in life circumstances or stressors to account for the clinical picture. Upon presenting to the clinic for neuropsychological evaluation, the primary complaint was that he was no longer able to read consistently or write fluently. In an effort to compensate and hide his deficits (i.e., he was embarrassed to admit to parents that he had not been wearing a helmet), he printed the alphabet, including arrows with each letter to remind him how to formulate the letters. This compensatory strategy was highly inefficient, and the post-concussive symptoms were brought to clinical attention. Neuropsychological testing revealed verbal and perceptual cognitive skills above the 90th percentile. Reading, spelling, and writing were impaired severely. Treatment results for this patient are presented in the next chapter.

Reducing Risk and Return-to-Play Issues

So, how do we reduce the risk to our sons/daughters, students, athletes, or patients of developing persistent post-concussion symptoms of the MIND subtype? The first, and most obvious, recommendations are education and prevention. Coaches, athletic trainers, parents, and the children themselves need to understand what a concussion is and what to do if a concussion has been sustained or is strongly suspected. Prevention also includes the regular use of proper protective gear, such as correctly fitting helmets.

Over the past decade, discussion has increased in the clinical literature regarding developing return-to-play guidelines in amateur sports (e.g., Cohen, Gioia, Atabaki, & Teach, 2009; Kirkwood, Yeates, & Wilson, 2006; Meehan & Bachur, 2009; Purcell, 2009). The eventual development of empirical guidelines hopefully will result in a rational basis for advising pediatric patients with mild TBI when they may safely resume physical activity and active participation in sport. One of the authors of this chapter, George Phillips, M.D., Associate Professor of Pediatrics at the University of Iowa Carver College of Medicine and the University of Iowa Children's Hospital, is a pediatrician who also is certified in pediatric sports medicine. Based upon existing data and his own experiences, Dr. Phillips (2008) has presented some clinical guidelines with regard to return-to-play. With one concussion, the child or adolescent should be taken out of play or competition until all symptoms have resolved and remained absent for at least 24 hours. This is the first step in a return-to-play protocol (Table 11–2). In spite of following such guidelines carefully, a small proportion of patients do not recover and are not able to progress along the steps of the return-to-play protocol. Early identification, evaluation, and appropriate treatment of those patients who experience persistent post-concussive symptoms are essential to reducing the burden of pediatric concussion.

Summary

Eighty to ninety percent of children who sustain a traumatic brain injury, experience a concussion or mild TBI. Most events of pediatric concussion occur during sports or at play, and the vast majority of those patients followed by Drs. Murph, Phillips, and

Table 11-2. Clinical Issues Regarding Return-to-Play for Children and Adolescents

- An athlete should return to play following a concussion only after being medically cleared to do so by a health-care provider.

- No concussed, young athlete should be permitted to return to play the same day as the concussion.

- No strenuous activity of any kind is recommended while the athlete is still symptomatic, including headaches.

- It is far more important to miss a game or a few practices than it is to miss out on a whole season or to live with the effects of a subsequent concussion.

- An athlete should be completely symptom free before returning to active practice or play.

- When the athlete becomes symptom-free, start out with light physical activity; if symptoms return with light activity, wait another 7–10 days before beginning with light activity once again.

- When the athlete is symptom-free with light activity, then he/she can progress to increased activity in a step-wise fashion.

- An inadvertent second impact (e.g., a subsequent concussion due to a fall) following the first impact *always* should be taken seriously and medically evaluated.

- The health-care provider also should check on the athlete's cognitive performance (e.g., ask about academic performance, check mental status, repeat ImPACT assessment, etc.) as well as inquiring about symptoms and motor coordination; if possible, compare current cognitive function with pre-participatory performance.

- Return-to-play decisions currently are made on an individual basis based upon variables such as previous history of concussion, severity of most recent concussion, age of athlete, gender of athlete, risk of future head impact (e.g., football versus golf).

Table 11-2. *continued*

> - It is generally better to err on the side of caution with return-to-play decisions; physical rest and informed reassurance are important contributors to resolution of symptoms in most cases.
>
> - With individualized management and step-wise return to physical activity, full recovery of function and remission of symptoms can be expected for the majority of child and adolescent athletes.
>
> - When assessing a patient for an acute concussion, always inquire about past history of concussion or head trauma.
>
> - Provide patient education regarding the recovery of function and future risk management (e.g., helmets when biking, using seatbelts).
>
> - Additional research on return-to-play guidelines for pediatric patients is needed.

Adapted from: Phillips, G. C. (2008). Update on concussion management. Grand Rounds presentation to the Department of Internal Medicine, Carver College of Medicine, University of Iowa, Iowa City.

M. A. Roberts have not involved litigation. A large majority of children who experience concussion (i.e., 70% to 85%) will recover fully by three months post-injury. Only a small proportion (i.e., 15% to 30%) will go on to have persistent symptoms of post-concussive dysfunction. Although symptoms such as staring spells, anger outbursts, tinnitus, or headache may occur only episodically, they can severely disrupt daily life at home and school. The first step in assessment of pediatric mild TBI is to identify whether a concussion has occurred. Several reasons have been described in the present chapter for failure to identify a concussion or for failure to associate the concussive event with the subsequent manifestation of clinical symptoms. Previous outcome research often has excluded all but those who have had a single, mild TBI. The conceptual framework of such research centers on two questions: (1) Does pediatric mild TBI, as a whole, result in persistent symptoms that demonstrate some recovery over time? and (2) If sequelae occur, how do the symptoms fit in with known categories of developmental disorders (e.g., psychopathology)?

We have suggested that a different sort of conceptual framework is necessary. Functional neuro-imaging evidence and neurophysiological research supports a neuro-electric explanation for failure to recover from pediatric mild TBI. Collateral sources of information (i.e., parents, guardians, teachers) also should be interviewed when children who experience persistent postconcussive disorder complain of episodic somatosensory, cognitive, and affective symptoms. It has been argued in Chapters 1 through 5, that such patients display an identifiable subtype of post-concussive disorder labeled MIND (i.e., Multiple Intermittent Neurobehavioral Disorder). Semistructured interview, symptom ratings, and typical findings from the neuropsychological assessment of children with the MIND subtype have been described. Prevention and return-to-play guidelines have been included. In the next chapter, treatment and outcome of the pediatric MIND subtype are presented.

References

Agrawal, D., Gowda, N. K., Bal, C. S., Pant, M., Mahapatra, A. K. (2005). Is medial temporal injury responsible for pediatric postconcussion syndrome? A prospective controlled study with single-photon emission computerized tomography. *Journal of Neurosurgery, 102*(Suppl. 2), 167–171.

American Psychiatric Association. (1994). *Diagnostic and statistical manual of mental disorders* (4th ed.). Washington, D.C.: Author.

Ayr, L. K., Yeates, K. O., Taylor, H. G., & Browne, M. (2009). Dimensions of postconcussive symptoms in children with mild traumatic brain injuries. *Journal of the International Neuropsychological Society, 15*(1), 19–30.

Benton, A. L., & Hamsher, K. (1989). *Multilingual Aphasia Exam* (2nd ed.). Iowa City, IA: AJA Associates.

Cohen, A. S., Pfister, B. J., Schwarzback, E., Grady, M. S., Goforth, P. B., & Satin, L. S. (2007). Injury-induced alterations in CNS electrophysiology. *Progress in Brain Research, 161,* 143–169.

Cohen, J. S., Gioia, G., Atabaki, S., & Teach, S. J. (2009). Sports-related concussions in pediatrics. *Current Opinion in Pediatrics, 21,* 288–293.

Dick, R. W. (2009). Is there a gender difference in concussion incidence and outcomes? *British Journal of Sports Medicine, 43*(Suppl. 1), 46–50.

Ewing-Cobbs, L., Levin, H. S., Fletcher, J. M., Miner, M. E., & Eisenberg, H. M. (1990). The Children's Orientation and Amnesia Test: Relationship to severity of acute head injury and to recovery of memory. *Neurosurgery, 27*(5), 683–691.

Fay, T. B., Yeates, K. O., Taylor, H. G., Bangert, B., Dietrich, A., Nuss, K. E., . . . Wright, M. (2010). Cognitive reserve as a moderator of postconcussion syndrome in children with complicated and uncomplicated mild traumatic brain injury. *Journal of the International Neuropsychological Society, 16,* 94–105.

Gerrard-Morris, A., Taylor, H. G., Yeates, K. O., Walz, N. C., Stancin, T., Minich, N., & Wade, S. L. (2010). Cognitive development after traumatic brain injury in young children. *Journal of the International Neuropsychological Society, 16*(1), 157–168.

Geyer, C., Ulrich, A., Gräfe, G., Stach, B., & Still, H. (2009). Diagnostic value of S100B and neuron-specific enolase in mild pediatric traumatic brain injury. *Journal of Neurosurgery. Pediatrics, 4*(4), 339–344.

Giza, C. C., & Hovda, D. A. (2001). The neurometabolic cascade of concussion. *Journal of Athletic Training, 36*(3), 228–235.

Gowda, N. K., Agrawal, D., Bal, C., Chandrashekar, N., Tripati, M., Bandopadhyaya, G. P., . . . Mahapatra, A. K. (2006). Technetium Tc-00m ethyl cysteinate dimmer brain single-photon emission CT in mild traumatic brain injury: A prospective study. *American Journal of Neuroradiology, 27*(2), 447–451.

Gronwall, D., Wrightson, P., & McGinn, V. (1997). Effect of mild head injury during the preschool years. *Journal of the International Neuropsychological Society, 3*(6), 592–597.

Guskiewicz, K. M., McCrea, M., Marshall, S. W., Cantu, R. C., Randolph, C., Barr, W., . . . Kelly, J. P. (2003). Cumulative effects associated with recurrent concussion in collegiate football players: The NCAA Concussion Study. *Journal of the American Medical Association, 290*(19), 2549–2555.

Kirkwood, M. W., Yeates, K. O., & Wilson, P. E. (2006). Pediatric sport-related concussion: a review of the clinical management of an oft-neglected population. *Pediatrics, 117,* 1359–1371.

Levin, H. S., Hanten, G., Roberson, G., Li, X., Ewing-Cobbs, L., Dennis, M., . . . Swank, P. (2008). Prediction of cognitive sequelae based on abnormal computed tomography findings in children following mild traumatic brain injury. *Journal of Neurosurgery. Pediatrics, 1*(6), 461–470.

Levin, H. S., Hanten, G., Zhang, L., Swank, P. R., Ewing-Cobbs, L., Dennis, M., . . . Hunter, J. V. (2004). Changes in working memory after traumatic brain injury in children. *Neuropsychology, 18*(2), 240–247.

Longhi, L., Saatman, K. E., Fujimoto, S., Raghupathi, R., Meaney, D. F., Davis, J., . . . McIntosh, T. K. (2005). Temporal window of vulnerability to repetitive experimental concussive brain injury. *Neurosurgery, 56*(2), 364–374.

Max, J. E., Lansing, A. E., Koele, S. L., Castillo, C. S., Bokura, H., Schachar, R., . . . Williams, K. E. (2004). Attention Deficit Hyperactivity Disorder in children and adolescents following traumatic brain injury. *Developmental Neuropsychology, 25*(1 & 2), 159–177.

McCrea, M., Hammeke, T., Olsen, G., Leo, P., & Guskiewicz, K. (2004). Unreported concussion in high school football players: implications for prevention. *Clinical Journal of Sport Medicine, 14*(1), 13–17.

Meehan, W. P., & Bachur, R. G. (2009). Sport-related concussion. *Pediatrics, 123,* 114–123.

Moran, L. M., Taylor, H. G., Ganesalingam, K., Gastier-Foster, J. M., Frick, J., Bangert, B., . . . Yeates, K. O. (2009). Apolipoprotein E4 as a predictor of outcome in mild traumatic brain injury. *Journal of Neurotrauma, 26*(9), 1489–1495.

Phillips, G. C. (2008). *Update on concussion management*. Grand Rounds presentation to the Department of Internal Medicine, Carver College of Medicine, University of Iowa, Iowa City, IA.

Piazza, A., Storti, M. P., Cotena, S., Stoppa, F., Perrotta, D., Esposito, G., . . . Tufano, R. (2007). S100B is not a reliable prognostic index in paediatric TBI. *Pediatric Neurosurgery, 43*(4), 258–264.

Ponsford, J., Willmott, C., Rothwell, A., Cameron, P., Ayton, G., Nelms, R., . . . Ng, R. T. (1999). Cognitive and behavioral outcome following mild traumatic injury in children. *Journal of Head Trauma Rehabilitation, 14*(4), 360–372.

Purcell, L. (2009). What are the most appropriate return to play guidelines for concussed child athletes? *British Journal of Sports Medicine, 43*, i51–i155.

Roberts, M. A. (1992). *The Pediatric Inventory of Neurobehavioral Symptoms (PINS)*. Iowa City, IA: University of Iowa.

Roberts, M. A. (1999). Mild traumatic brain injury in children and adolescents. In N. R. Varney, & R. J. Roberts, (Eds.), *Mild head injury: Causes, evaluation, and treatment* (pp. 493–512). Mahwah, NJ: Lawrence Erlbaum Associates.

Roberts, M. A. (2006). *Persistent post-concussion syndrome: What are the risks?* Iowa Department of Education Traumatic Brain Injury Project. Iowa Communications Network: University of Iowa.

Roberts, M. A., & Furuseth, A. (1997). Eliciting parental report following pediatric traumatic brain injury: Preliminary findings on the Pediatric Inventory of Neurobehavioral Symptoms. *Archives of Clinical Neuropsychology, 12*, 449–457.

Roberts, M. A., Manshadi, F. F., Bushnell, D. L., & Hines, M. E. (1995). Neurobehavioral dysfunction following mild traumatic brain injury in childhood: A case report with positive findings on positron emission tomography. *Brain Injury, 9*, 427–436.

Roberts, M. A., Persinger, M. A., Grote, C., Evertowski, L. M., Springer, J. A., Tuten, J., . . . Baglio, C. S. (1994). The Dichotic Word Listening Test: Preliminary observations in American and Canadian samples. *Applied Neuropsychology, 1*, 45–56.

Roberts, M. A., Verduyn, W. H., Manshadi, F. F., & Hines, M. E. (1996). Episodic symptoms in dysfunctioning children and adolescents following mild and severe traumatic brain injury. *Brain Injury, 10,* 739–747.

Roberts, M. A., Wright, S. E., & Roberts, R. J. (2006). *Post-concussive symptoms in a pediatric population: The importance of what we ask, whom we ask, and when we ask it.* Poster presentation at the Annual Meeting of the International Neuropsychological Society, Chicago, IL.

Roberts, R. J. (1999). Epilepsy Spectrum Disorder in the context of mild traumatic brain injury. In N. R. Varney, & R. J. Roberts, (Eds.), *Mild head injury: Causes, evaluation, and treatment* (pp. 209–247). Mahwah, NJ: Lawrence Erlbaum Associates.

Roberts, R. J., Gorman, L. L., Lee, G. P., Hines, M. E., Richardson, E. D., Riggle, T. A., & Varney, N. R. (1992). The phenomenology of multiple partial seizure-like symptoms without stereotyped spells: An epilepsy spectrum disorder? *Epilepsy Research, 13*(2), 167–177.

Roberts, R. J., Springer, J. A., & Roberts, M. A. (1990). *Dichotic Word Listening Test—English Version.* St Louis, MO: Auditec of St. Louis.

Sattler, J. M. (2006). *Assessment of Children: behavioral, social, and clinical foundations.* San Diego, CA: J.M. Sattler.

Sattler, J. M. (2002). *Assessment of Children: behavioral and clinical applications.* San Diego, CA: J.M. Sattler.

Satz, P. (1993). Brain reserve capacity on symptom onset after brain injury: A formulation and review of evidence for threshold theory. *Neuropsychology, 7,* 273–295.

Schatz, P., Pardini, J. E., Lovell, M. R., Collins, M. W., & Podell, K. (2006). Sensitivity and specificity of the ImPACT Test Battery for concussion in athletes. *Archives of Clinical Neuropsychology, 21,* 91–99.

Shaw, N. A. (2002). The neurophysiology of concussion. *Progress in Neurobiology, 67*(4), 281–344.

Taylor, D. C., & Lochery, M. (1987). Temporal lobe epilepsy: Origin and significance of simple and complex auras. *Journal of Neurology, Neurosurgery, & Psychiatry, 50,* 673-681.

Taylor, H. G., Dietrich, A., Nuss, K., Wright, M., Rusin, J., Bangert, B., . . . Yeates, K .O. (2010). Post-concussive symptoms in children with mild traumatic brain injury. *Neuropsychology,* 24(2), 148–159.

Theriault, M., DeBeaumont, L., Tremblay, S., Lassonde, M., & Jolicoeur, P. (May 17, 2010). Cumulative effects of concussions in athletes revealed by electrophysiological abnormalities on visual working memory. *Journal of Clinical & Experimental Neuropsychology,* 1–12 [epub ahead of print].

Umile, E. M., Sandel, M. E., Alavi, A., Terry, C. M., & Plotkin, R. C. (2002). Dynamic Imaging in mild traumatic brain injury: Support for the theory of medial temporal vulnerability. *Archives of Physical Medicine and Rehabilitation, 83,* 1506–1513.

Vagnozzi, R., Signoretti, S., Tavazzi, B., Floris, R., Lucovici, A., Marziali, S., . . . Lazzarino, G. (2008). Temporal Windows of metabolic brain vulnerability to concussion: A pilot 1H-magnetic resonance spectroscopic study in concussed athletes—part III. *Neurosurgery, 62*(6), 1286–1295.

Wrightson, P., McGinn, V., & Gronwall, D. (1995). Mild head injury in preschool children: Evidence that it can be associated with a persistent cognitive deficit. *Journal of Neurology, Neurosurgery, & Psychiatry, 59*(4), 375–380.

Yeates, K. O., & Taylor, H. G. (2005). Neurobehavioural outcomes of mild head injury in children and adolescents. *Pediatric Rehabilitation, 8*(1), 5–16.

Yeates, K. O., Taylor, H. G., Rusin, J., Bangert, B., Dietrich, A., Nuss, K., . . . Jones, B. L. (2009). Longitudinal trajectories of postconcussive symptoms in children with mild traumatic brain injuries and their relationship to acute clinical status. *Pediatrics, 123*(3), 735–743.

Yu, Z., & Morrison, B. (2010). Experimental mild traumatic brain injury induces functional alteration of the developing hippocampus. *Journal of Neurophysiology, 103,* 499–510.

12

Pediatric Mild TBI, Episodic Symptoms, and Treatment Considerations

. . . In the hippocampus, research now suggests that TBI regionally alters the delicate balance between excitatory and inhibitory neurotransmission in surviving neurons, disrupting the normal functioning of synaptic circuits . . . and how these alterations contribute to cognitive impairment and a reduction in seizure threshold associated with human concussive brain injury.

—Akiva Cohen, et al. (2007, p.143)

Introduction

Subtyping of children with persistent post-concussive symptoms has been proposed as a means of advancing our understanding of causes and proposing new and effective treatments (Taylor et al., 2010) for this disorder. Taylor, Yeates, and colleagues (Ayr,

Yeates, Taylor, & Browne, 2009; Taylor et. al., 2010) suggested a focus on individual symptoms that are *unique* to persistent post-concussive disorder when compared to symptoms associated with other traumatic injuries.

In the previous chapter on assessment of post-concussive symptoms following pediatric mild traumatic brain injury, the MIND subtype was described. M.A. Roberts's previous research (Roberts, M. A., 1999; Roberts, Wright, & Roberts, 2006) pointed out the importance of the method by which the assessment is conducted. It is essential to acknowledge the importance of *whom* we ask, *what* we ask, and *when* we ask questions about post-concussive symptoms.

In a study of pediatric, mild TBI (see Roberts, M. A., 1999), the Iowa Interview was administered to parents of matched groups of children and adolescents with orthopedic injury or mild traumatic brain injury. Parents of the children with ortho-pedic injuries reported a zero-percent incidence rate of the four most common episodic symptoms (i.e., anger outbursts, staring spells, tinnitus, and headaches). Parents of the children with a single mild TBI event (i.e., who were selected as consecutive referrals to hospital emergency treatment centers and who also matched the orthopedic subjects on demographics) reported a 12% incidence rate of the four most common episodic symp-toms. This 12% rate of MIND symptoms is slightly lower than the 15% to 30% estimate of pediatric post-concussive symptoms, suggesting that the pediatric patients with MIND symptoms may indeed be a subtype of pediatric post-concussive disorder. A third comparison group (Roberts & Simcox, 1996) of children referred for medical and neuropsychological evaluation follow-ing failure to recover from mild TBI also was provided in M. A. Roberts' (1999) chapter. Parents of referred pediatric patients reported that 92% of their children displayed the four most com-mon MIND symptoms. This finding suggests that the MIND subtype possibly may make up a large proportion of those chil-dren and adolescents who fail to recover from mild TBI. Inde-pendent replication of these findings is recommended, given the level of controversy regarding the topic of mild TBI in general.

In the present book, we propose reconsideration of episodic, post-concussive symptoms (i.e., labeled with the acronym MIND, explained throughout the book) as a valid subtype of persistent post-concussive disorder for children, adolescents, and adults. The symptoms have been described as Epilepsy Spectrum Disorder (Roberts, R. J., et al., 1992), and neuroimaging results (Agrawal, Gowda, Bal, Pant, & Mahapatra, 2005; Gowda et al., 2006) in children have documented post-concussive symptoms associated with temporal lobe hypo-perfusion during the acute period, as well as at three months post-injury. Given the parallels of the MIND subtype with episodic mood disorders and partial complex seizures, open medication trials of treatment with a mood stabilizer with anticonvulsant properties, such as carbamazepine and valproic acid, are likely to be beneficial (Roberts, Verduyn, Manshadi, & Hines, 1996). Anecdotally, we also have observed clinical success in treating some patients for short periods of time with levetiracetam (Bootsma et al., 2007; Cereghino et al., 2000; Stoner, Lea, Wolf, & Berges, 2005).

In children and adolescents, there are no placebo-controlled studies of these medication treatments in mild TBI. However, a series of open trial case studies (Roberts, Manshadi, Bushnell, & Hines, 1995; Roberts, Verduyn, Manshadi, & Hines, 1996) reported that most pediatric patients with persistent post-concussive disorder experienced a good to excellent treatment outcome with either carbamazepine or valproic acid. In this book, we have proposed testable hypotheses regarding potential medical treatments for the MIND subtype. Independent, controlled research, using placebo and active medications, with random assignment of subjects, blinded interviews, and neuropsychological testing, needs to be conducted.

First Pediatric Case Study

Let us return now to the young man described in the pediatric assessment chapter who had experienced two blunt force traumas to the back, left quadrant of the skull within less than a month's time. Although he had been an excellent student, after the second injury, he could no longer read or write fluently and was experiencing disabling headaches. He required significant academic accommodations including a shortened school day, reduced assignments, and open-book, untimed exams. These accommodations, although necessary for the completion of any school work, did not address the underlying cause of the persistent post-concussive MIND symptoms. Rather, these adjustments at school provided only temporary compensatory strategies for this young man. Magnetic Resonance Imaging (i.e., MRI, which examines structural brain integrity) was normal. After the neuropsychological and medical evaluations, this patient was treated with carbamazepine and followed by the chapter authors. At one-month follow-up, the patient was decidedly improved and could attend school full days with only minor headaches. After two months of treatment with carbamazepine, the patient had recovered to his previous advanced level of reading and writing fluency. This young man was continued on carbamazepine for an additional 6 months, after which he was tapered off, and the medication was discontinued. Post-concussive symptoms did not recur. This case exemplifies our collective clinical treatment experience with children and teens who do not fully recover following mild TBI: often, the sooner the medication treatment is initiated following symptom onset, the quicker the resolution of symptoms; thus, the overall treatment period is generally shorter.

A Second Pediatric Case Study

A second case initially presented as a diagnostic conundrum. A boy attending middle school was admitted to a tertiary care hospital during the late summer months, after local and regional medical care was unsuccessful in addressing this boy's neurologic symptoms. Essentially, this right-handed boy abruptly developed intermittent expressive and receptive aphasia. Between episodes, he was able to speak and comprehend normally. He originally was diagnosed as being dehydrated, as he had been participating in football practice during the hottest days of the summer. Rehydration was unsuccessful in alleviating his acute symptoms, and the patient went on to experience more frequent episodes of aphasia. Neurologic work-up at the tertiary-care medical center was negative. In response to the Iowa Interview, the boy and his parents reported a high frequency (score well above the 95th percentile for children) of episodic MIND symptoms. Also, during the interview, the boy responded to some questions in a clear fashion, but often digressed during his responses to uttering nonmeaningful speech. Scores on the Multi-Lingual Aphasia Exam (Benton & Hamsher, 1989) were at the first percentile for Visual Naming, Verbal Fluency, Sentence Repetition, and the Token Test. Employing gestures along with verbal instructions, the boy was able to score in only the average range on selected Perceptual Reasoning subtests from the Wechsler Intelligence Scale for Children-IV (Wechsler, 2003). This boy had an A grade-point average prior to the onset of the current aphasic symptoms. Extended history information was obtained from parents and revealed a negative history for early childhood illness or head trauma. However, when queried about the one month prior to the onset of symptoms, the boy's parents reported two events of blunt-force trauma during football practice. Both blows to the head were to the left anterior quadrant, with the second event a helmet-to-helmet hit with another player. The boy was somewhat dazed after the second blow, but he began to feel better after he sat on the sidelines for a short time drinking fluids. Once home from practice, he began to manifest some unusual speech. Family members later noted a dent in the left front portion of his helmet. This patient was started on carbamazepine while still hospitalized. At six weeks outpatient follow-up, the boy's parents reported treatment to be a resounding success, indicating that they were "thrilled to have their son back." Neuropsychological testing results on the Multi-Lingual Aphasia Exam were now within normal limits. Once again, this child did not require extended medical treatment, and by one year post-injury had completely and successfully been able to discontinue medication treatment.

A Third Pediatric Case Study

In a third case, the symptom presentation also included significant emotional post-concussive symptoms. Christopher, a popular 5th grade student, had just been elected to the school's Student Council from his class. During the summer months prior to the start of school, Christopher had fallen while running and hit the back of his head on concrete. Although there were no witnesses and Christopher had amnesia for the event, his parents were nearby, and given the short time span involved, it seemed unlikely that he sustained a loss of consciousness. He recovered quickly, had no visible trauma, other than a minor abrasion and bruise on the back of his head. He was not taken for medical evaluation because of the perceived minor nature of the accident. Five days later, Christopher was lifting a bicycle from an overhead rack when his grip slipped, with the bicycle striking him on the top frontal area of the head (i.e., the vertex). He was bleeding, dazed, and confused, as he walked into the house. Christopher had amnesia for the event and for a period of time prior to, and immediately following, the event. He appeared to be confused, and although he recognized family members, he did not remember where he was; nor could he recall the name of his favorite pet. He was evaluated by his pediatrician, had no localizing neurologic signs, but continued to appear confused during the examination. A brain CT scan was performed, which was unremarkable. Parents were instructed to observe carefully for any changes and to call or return for medical attention if there were concerns. His parents were reassured and assumed that their child had escaped a potentially serious brain injury. Once again, Christopher seemed to have recovered from this second blunt force trauma. However, Christopher continued to experience moderate headaches that recurred intermittently for many months.

Within weeks of the second head injury, Christopher also began experiencing difficulties in "automatic wandering." This was manifested by new behaviors that had not been seen previously: riding his bike long distances into the country and not returning until after dark; going to a friend's house in the neighborhood without permission and staying for several hours without calling parents or returning home. Because of parental concerns, the police were called on at least three occasions when he wandered away and could not be found. When he was returned home, Christopher seemed relatively oblivious to the reasons for adult concern and surprised by the distress of the adults around him. He also had no perception of how long he had been absent on any of the occasions. Christopher was reported not to be angry or depressed, and he never lied about where he was, what he was doing, or whom he was with. The reader will recall that this type of "automatic wandering" is similar to one of the post-concussive symptoms of MIND and an item on the Iowa Interview for adults (Roberts, R. J., 1999).

When school started in the fall, Christopher began experiencing difficulties almost immediately. Academically, his memory was poor, and his attention span and problems with distractibility were very pronounced. The stimulant medication dosage prescribed for previously diagnosed Attention-Deficit/Hyperactivity Disorder was no longer sufficient to improve his concentration. Over time, the stimulant dosage was increased to a maximum of 108 mg Concerta in the morning and 10 mg short-acting methylphenidate after school.

In addition to what appeared to be a remarkable worsening of his ADHD symptoms, Christopher also experienced a low tolerance for frustration, volatile moods with explosive outbursts, interpersonal difficulties with peers, and a change in personality. Christopher's school situation suddenly became a full-blown crisis, when he abruptly punched his best friend with no apparent provocation, knocking him to the blacktop during the noon lunch break. At home, he suddenly would become agitated with little provocation, lash out physically without warning toward family members, or throw objects or furniture.

This unpredictable violence, moodiness, and the remarkably worsened ADHD symptoms prompted Christopher's pediatrician, who was managing his care following the two concussive episodes (Kaye, Gallagher, Callahan, & Nance, 2010) to seek further evaluation by a child psychiatrist and child neurologist. A brain MRI and EEG were interpreted as normal, and Christopher was diagnosed with a cognitive disorder and Oppositional Defiant Disorder. This patient was followed by the child psychiatrist who prescribed a variety of medications, primarily atypical antipsychotics such as risperidone and olanzapine, but with little success. Paxil, an SSRI antidepressant, was helpful for the symptoms of anxiety, but did little for the sudden-onset mood changes and behavioral symptoms that were most problematic. Parents continued to report unpredictable, out-of-character explosive events, including a remarkable episode during a family vacation. Upon arrival at the hotel, Christopher became enraged when the zipper on his suitcase got stuck and he was unable to retrieve his swimming suit. He began yelling and throwing things around the room, causing enough of a disturbance that other guests asked that the desk clerk call to inquire whether the family needed assistance from the police or a social worker.

When referred for further medical and neuropsychological evaluation, the history of two closely spaced blunt-force traumas was obtained as a possible cause for the abrupt change in Christopher's behavior. Because both head injuries had been considered minor, Christopher was never hospitalized. His head imaging studies were unremarkable, and he seemed to recover from the initial event. Thus, neither the parents, nor the pediatrician, nor the psychiatrist considered that there might be a relationship between the two concussions that had occurred months earlier and the problematic, episodic behaviors Christopher manifested. As the present authors had been involved with his psychological and medical care for treatment of Attention-Deficit/Hyperactivity Disorder prior to the head traumas, these sudden changes were believed to be related to the concussive events.

Importantly, the results of testing completed prior to the TBI were available for comparison with evaluations performed following the injury. Significant declines were evident in verbal and visual reasoning skills, verbal fluency and memory—including immediate and delayed recall of verbal information and immediate visual memory. Christopher also had difficulty organizing and generating information. A test of dichotic word listening (Roberts, Springer, & Roberts, 1990), which previously had been normal, showed an abnormally low score for repeating words presented to the left auditory channel. As noted in the preceding chapter on assessment of pediatric patients, the finding of a dichotic word listening abnormality is highly predictive of the MIND subtype of persistent post-concussive disorder.

At this point, it became clear that Christopher's somatic complaint of persistent headaches; his academic problems with language, memory, and attention; as well as his extreme behavioral and mood changes could be explained by the diagnosis of post-concussion syndrome. The correct diagnosis led to the initiation of effective treatment. In this case, treatment with carbamazepine (Tegretol) was initiated and slowly increased to optimize clinical improvement. Within weeks, parents began to report striking improvement in mood and behavior. Christopher experienced improved frustration tolerance, fewer altercations with peers, and more positive interactions at home and school. As the carbamazepine dose was optimized, Christopher returned to school and no longer demonstrated the abrupt outbursts that brought him to medical attention.

Christopher continued to be followed clinically by the chapter authors over several years. He tested to be a very bright young man with cognitive scores at, or above, the 95th percentile. Christopher enrolled in college and maintained his medical regimen (i.e., stimulant and carbamazepine) during his freshman year living in the dormitory. By his sophomore year in college, Christopher rented an apartment with friends. He did not maintain the same structured routine he had while in the dormitory and began to intermittently forget to take his medications. His school performance declined; he became forgetful, often not recalling class lectures; and he became even more disorganized. Although he had done well academically during his freshman year, during his sophomore year Christopher was failing most of his classes. Medication treatment was re-initiated, first with stimulant medication and then with carbamazepine. After a review of his academic credentials and medical history with student services at his college, Christopher again returned to earning above average course grades. Although diagnosed shortly after the onset of symptoms, in Christopher's case, he required ongoing treatment with medication over the years in order to be successful academically.

Considerations Regarding Younger Children

Diagnosis and treatment of very young children with the MIND subtype of post-concussion disorder can be quite difficult. Young children have a more limited history of stable baseline behavioral or cognitive development. Typically developing children in the 4- to 7-year-old age range manifest behavior stages (e.g., temper tantrums) that generally are transitory with appropriate behavior management strategies. Careful history and observation of the child during testing or play may lead the examiner to support or disconfirm the diagnosis of post-concussive disorder. Extended experience with child developmental stages is exceedingly important. During neuropsychological evaluations, the examiner may observe staring spells. When observing play, abrupt mood changes without provocation may support the association with previous concussion. Also, the young child's preschool or kindergarten teacher presumably has had experience with many same-age peers and may be able to shed light on any changes that have been observed.

Communication of Treatment Recommendations to Local Care Providers

In distant areas of rural states such as Iowa and Minnesota, the actual treatment of many patients likely is to be initiated or managed by care providers with generalist practices (e.g., pediatrics, family practice, internal medicine) rather than by specialists (e.g., neurologists, psychiatrists, sports medicine physicians, physiatrists) who tend to practice in more populous urban areas. When such is the case, it is important to be clear and fairly detailed about treatment recommendations to the local care provider who ultimately will be responsible for electing to treat a patient with MIND-like symptoms on an ongoing basis.

Providing a brief, but clear summary of the recommended medication plan can be helpful in promoting positive outcomes. A sample medication plan for a 17-year-old patient whose local family practice physician practices in a remote, rural area is presented in Table 12–1.

Table 12-1. Sample Medication Plan for an Adolescent Sports Medicine Patient with MIND

Dear Dr. X:

Thank you for referring your 17-year-old, patient *Y* for evaluation. Patient Y has experienced multiple concussions, each of which resulted in significant symptoms that lasted beyond the typical 7-to-10-day course of recovery for "simple" (i.e., uncomplicated) sports-concussion. As part of our evaluation, formal neuropsychological testing indicated persistent decline in short-term, verbal memory functioning. Objective decline in school grades also has been observed since patient *Y*'s most recent concussion. According to the patient's parents and school personnel, despite good effort on the part of the patient to study for tests and get homework completed, his grades have declined. In addition, the patient and his family report the development of multiple episodic symptoms (e.g., frequent headaches, memory gaps, participating in unrecalled conversations, ringing in the ears, pointless temper outbursts with little if any provocation). These symptoms started following the most recent concussion.

continues

Table 12-1. *continued*

This constellation of intermittent symptoms often is indicative of a subtype of post-concussive syndrome termed an "epilepsy spectrum disorder" by neuro-psychiatrists in the 1990s. Currently, my colleagues and I have used the less controversial acronym MIND (for Multiple Intermittent Neurobehavioral Disorder) to identify patients with this subtype of persistent post-concussive, clinical presentation. Although presently no randomized clinical trials of treatment for such patients are available, numerous case reports and case series from multiple researchers and clinicians, both here and abroad, have documented similar symptom clusters and persistent, neuro-cognitive impairments and complaints in patients following seemingly mild traumatic brain injury.

The proposed mechanism for this condition possibly may be due to a focus of injury sending inappropriate neuro-electric signals to other areas of the brain, resulting in a so-called "kindling effect" that leads to such intermittent symptoms and cognitive difficulties. Such symptoms are similar to those of partial seizure disorders, but MIND patients usually have normal EEG findings or nonspecific changes on EEG. When obtained, structural neuro-imaging results are also typically unremarkable. In several case series, patients experienced worsening symptoms on medications that are known to lower seizure threshold, but improved with anti-epileptic medications, such as carbamazepine, which actively raise seizure threshold.

At our specialty clinic, we have followed a number of patients with this condition, and we have experienced considerable success with the use of carbamazepine, typically at maintenance doses of 600 mg/day. Patient Y reportedly has experienced noticeable, clinical improvement in his symptoms, by his account and his parents' account. His memory and processing abilities also have improved somewhat, since starting on carbamazepine 2 months ago.

Because patient Y's insurance does not cover the extended-release form that we use typically, patient Y was started on 200 mg. of carbamazepine once a day for one

Table 12-1. *continued*

week, followed by 200 mg. b.i.d. for one week, and patient *Y* is now on 300 mg. b.i.d. for maintenance. Attached are baseline lab values for CBC with diff., BUN/Cr, and liver function tests.

It was explained to patient *Y* and his family that he does not have a traditional form of epilepsy, even though he takes a medication that often is prescribed for patients with conventional seizure disorders. He does not have restrictions on his activities that patients with epilepsy might have, such as driving. He was told to refrain from playing varsity football this coming season, however, due to the risk of another concussion. He most likely does not need to have carbamazepine levels drawn to assess efficacy of treatment compared to some targeted therapeutic range. He should be followed with office visits every 2–3 months, and he probably should have the preceding blood-work drawn at those times within the first 5–6 months of ongoing treatment.

Our general experience has been that the medication is well-tolerated and that patients such as Y generally do well when treated with such medication for about a year. Then, if the previous intermittent symptoms remain well-controlled, we typically attempt to wean patients off this medication using a 2–3 week taper. If symptoms noticeably increase during such a taper, the patient should be returned to his maintenance dose and stabilized there for another 2–3 months before attempting another taper. Typically our patients have had improvement with intermittent psycho-sensory and affective symptoms within the first few weeks of maintenance treatment, and then improvement in cognitive processing later in the 2–3 month trial. However, some residual symptoms may remain, even when treatment is deemed to be optimal.

Thank you for this interesting referral, and please do not hesitate to contact me as circumstances warrant. After school resumes, please do not hesitate to contact our clinical neuropsychologist *Z* if problems with educational performance become apparent.

References

Agrawal, D., Gowda, N. K., Bal, C. S., Pant, M., & Mahapatra, A. K. (2005). Is medial temporal injury responsible for pediatric postconcussion syndrome? A prospective controlled study with single-photon emission computerized tomography. *Journal of Neurosurgery, 102*(Suppl. 2), 167–171.

Ayr, L. K., Yeates, K. O., Taylor, H. G., & Browne, M. (2009). Dimensions of postconcussive symptoms in children with mild traumatic brain injuries. *Journal of the International Neuropsychological Society, 15*(1), 19–30.

Benton, A. L., & Hamsher, K. deS. (1989). *Multilingual Aphasia Exam* (2nd ed.). Iowa City, IA: AJA Associates.

Bootsma, H. P. R., Ricker, L., Diepman, L., Gehring, J., Hulsman, J., Lambrechts, D., . . . Aldenkamp, A. P. (2007). Levetiracetam in clinical practice: Long-term experience in patients with refractory epilepsy referred to a tertiary epilepsy center. *Epilepsy & Behavior, 10,* 296–303.

Cereghino, J. J., Biton, V., Abou-Khalil, B., Dreifuss, F., Gauer, L. J., & Leppik, I. (2000). Levetiracetam for partial seizures: Results of a double-blind, randomized clinical trial. *Neurology, 55*(2), 236–242.

Cohen, A. S., Pfister, B. J., Schwarzback, E., Grady, M. S., Goforth, P. B., & Satin, L. S. (2007). Injury-induced alterations in CNS electrophysiology. *Progress in Brain Research, 161,* 143–169.

Gowda, N. K., Agrawal, D., Bal, C., Chandrashekar, N., Tripati, M., Bandopadhyaya, G. P., . . . Mahapatra, A. K. (2006). Technetium Tc-00m ethyl cysteinate dimmer brain single-photon emission CT in mild traumatic brain injury: A prospective study. *American Journal of Neuroradiology, 27*(2), 447–451.

Kaye, A. J., Gallagher, R., Callahan, J. M., & Nance, M. L. (2010). Mild traumatic brain injury in the pediatric population: The role of the pediatrician in routine follow-up. *The Journal of Trauma® Injury, Infection, and Critical Care, 68*(6), 1396–1400.

Roberts, M. A. (1999). Mild traumatic brain injury in children and adolescents. In N. R. Varney & R. J. Roberts (Eds.), *Mild head injury: Causes, evaluation, and treatment* (pp. 493–512). Mahwah, NJ: Lawrence Erlbaum Associates.

Roberts, M. A., Manshadi, F. F., Bushnell, D. L., & Hines, M. E. (1995). Neurobehavioral dysfunction following mild traumatic brain injury in childhood: A case report with positive findings on positron emission tomography. *Brain Injury, 9,* 427–436.

Roberts, M. A., & Simcox, A. F. (1996). Assessing olfaction following pediatric traumatic brain injury. *Applied Neuropsychology, 3,* 86–88.

Roberts, M. A., Verduyn, W. H., Manshadi, F. F., & Hines, M. E. (1996). Episodic symptoms in dysfunctioning children and adolescents following mild and severe traumatic brain injury. *Brain Injury, 10,* 739–747.

Roberts, M. A., Wright, S. E., & Roberts, R. J. (2006). *Post-concussive symptoms in a pediatric population: The importance of what we ask, whom we ask, and when we ask it.* Poster presentation at the Annual Meeting of the International Neuropsychological Society, Chicago, IL.

Roberts, R. J. (1999). Epilepsy Spectrum Disorder in the context of mild traumatic brain injury. In N. R. Varney & R. J. Roberts (Eds.), *Mild head injury: Causes, evaluation, and treatment* (pp. 209–247). Mahwah, NJ: Lawrence Erlbaum Associates.

Roberts, R. J., Gorman, L. L., Lee, G. P., Hines, M. E., Richardson, E. D., Riggle, T. A., & Varney, N. R. (1992). The phenomenology of multiple partial seizure-like symptoms without stereotyped spells: An epilepsy spectrum disorder? *Epilepsy Research, 13*(2), 167–177.

Roberts, R. J., Springer, J. A., & Roberts, M. A. (1990). *Dichotic Word Listening Test—English version.* St. Louis, MO: Auditec of St. Louis.

Stoner, S. C., Lea, J. W., Wolf, A. L, & Berges, A. A. (2005). Levetiracetam for mood stabilization and maintenance of seizure control following multiple treatment failures. *The Annals of Pharmacotherapy, 39,* 1928–1931.

Taylor, D. C., & Moira, L. (1987). Temporal lobe epilepsy: Origin and significance of simple and complex auras. Journal of Neurology, Neurosurgery, and Psychiatry, 50, 673–681.

Taylor, H. G., Dietrich, A., Nuss, K., Wright, M., Rusin, J., Bangert, B., . . . Yeates, K. O. (2010). Post-concussive symptoms in children with mild traumatic brain injury. *Neuropsychology, 24*(2), 148–159.

Wechsler, D. (2003). *Wechsler Intelligence Scale for Children—Fourth edition.* San Antonio, TX: Pearson/Psychological Corporation.

13

Unanswered Questions and Issues Requiring Further Study

Curiosity comes from gaps in our knowledge.
— Chip Heath and Dan Heath (2007, p.90)

Is MIND Likely To Be a Genetic, Congenital, or Acquired Syndrome?

A genetic disorder is one whose expression is more or less programmed at conception. A common example of a highly heritable neurobehavioral disorder would be Huntington's disease. If a person is unfortunate enough to have the wrong combination of genes, they will almost certainly develop Huntington's disease. A congenital disorder is one that is present at birth, whether or not it is genetically based. An acquired disorder develops, either acutely or abruptly, over the course of one's life due predominantly to environmental factors.

We believe that the bulk of the evidence points to MIND being an acquired neurobehavioral disorder, one that is caused by damage or dysfunction in the brain due to certain types of physical trauma, most prominently blunt-force head trauma (Roberts, 1999). We also believe that other forms of acquired brain damage or dysfunction due to other causes (e.g., hypoxic damage, febrile damage, certain forms of toxic damage, blast exposure) can create a MIND-like clinical picture; however, in most industrialized nations, the most frequent cause is likely to be blunt-force trauma, such as that sustained with head trauma due to motor vehicle accidents and falls. [This is not necessarily the case for all industrialized countries; for example, as recently as 1986, the main cause of traumatic brain injury in the People's Republic of China was bicycle accidents (Wang et al., 1986).] That having been said, it seems highly likely that individual brains vary genetically (Loscher, 2009), or experientially (Kutcher & Eckner, 2010; Statler, Swank, Abildskov, Bigler, & White, 2008), with regard to susceptibility to developing post-traumatic symptoms of MIND.

We cannot rule out, however, that some congenital defects may be responsible occasionally for producing a MIND-like clinical picture. For instance, over the course of about 20 years, the second author has seen a series of 10 pediatric patients with negative histories for head trauma who experienced multiple, intermittent symptoms associated with paroxysmal theta bursts on EEG (M. A. Roberts, unpublished observations).

However, we suspect that the frequency of possible congenital MIND-like presentations most likely is extremely small in comparison to the number of children who experience multiple, episodic symptoms following blunt-force head trauma.

What Causes MIND?

At present, the precise cause (or causes) underlying the development of MIND remain to be elucidated. Based on the previous material covered in this book, it should be apparent that MIND (as a subtype of Persistent Post-Concussive Disorder) likely will prove to be a controversial diagnosis in the subfields of neuro-psychiatry and neuropsychology. Thus, it might seem premature for us to speculate upon the etiology of MIND in the book where we are proposing an operational diagnosis of the condition; however, we believe that it is "better to light one candle than to curse the darkness." We also realize that much research will be required on normal brain function, in addition to studies on abnormal brain function following blunt-force trauma, before the causes of MIND can be specified with certainty.

So we proceed cautiously, offering our collective specula-tions and hypotheses, ones that may well exceed the current knowledge base at times. At the present time, the most likely hypothesis is that the symptoms of MIND reflect underlying, subclinical, electrophysiological dysfunction in the brain.

What Is Meant by "Subclinical Electrophysiological Dysfunction?"

"Subclinical electrophysiological dysfunction" means that some brain structures or pools of neurons fire in an abnormally syn-chronized fashion, but that this electrical activity is not sufficiently widespread to produce an overt seizure. Subclinical electrical discharges or "subclinical seizures" may or may not be evident on standard EEG recordings. Put another way, a normal EEG recorded from the surface of the scalp does not rule out that small, but abnormal, electrophysiological responses may be occur-ring in deeper brain structures (Taylor, 1999). Studies of patients with electrodes actually implanted in brain tissues have revealed that abnormal electrical responses can occur in fairly large areas of the brain in the absence of apparent changes during standard EEG recordings from the outer surface of the skull (Wieser, Hail-ermariam, Regard, & Landis, 1985).

Considerable indirect evidence reveals that the basis of the proposed subgroup of patients with MIND may be due to "sub-clinical" electrical discharges in the brain, which are insufficient to produce a traditional epileptic seizure. The individual arguments are reviewed in the following list:

- MIND appears to respond favorably to medications that raise seizure-threshold (such as anticonvulsants) and respond poorly to medications that lower seizure threshold (Roberts, 1999; Tucker, Price, Johnson, & McAllister, 1986). These pharmacological responses are not logically sufficient to prove that underlying electrophysiological dysfunction is responsible for MIND; however, these observations are quite consistent with that possibility. Some authorities claim that anticonvulsant medications such as valproic acid and carbamazepine likely possess "psychotropic" properties that are separate from their anticonvulsant properties.

- Although patients with MIND-like symptoms following mild-to-moderate TBI typically do not produce clearly epileptiform EEGs from surface recordings, the frequency of any type of EEG abnormality clearly exceeds that found in a large-scale study of general psychiatric patients (Bridgers, 1988; R. J. Roberts, 1999).

- Both MIND patients and patients with conventional partial seizure disorders frequently fail dichotic word listening tasks (Roberts, Varney, Paulsen, & Richardson, 1990; Grote et al. 1995; Lee et al., 1994) in the absence of structural lesions on CT or MRI scans. This type of failure likely represents a type of electrical disconnection syndrome due to "neural noise" (Hutt, 1972).

- Individuals with TBI are at increased risk for developing both post-traumatic epilepsy (Agrawal, Timothy, Pandit, & Manju, 2006) and mood disorders (Jorge & Starkstein, 2005). Logically, it would seem that patients with TBI also would be at increased risk for MIND, which combines some of the features of conventional epilepsy and with some of the features of conventional mood disorders, but appears to be a distinctly diagnosable clinical entity in its own right.

How Does Such Subclinical Electrophysiological Activity Develop?

The truth is that no definitive answer can be provided at this time. However, *at least* four major mechanisms drawn from epilepsy research may prove to be relevant in the future: (a) kindling; (b) deafferentation; (c) the "hippocampal" model; and (d) so-called "pre-ictal" changes in neuronal function (i.e., those changes immediately preceding the onset of a conventionally defined seizure). These respective models are discussed in the order they are listed here. It should be emphasized that aspects of these various models are not necessarily mutually exclusive, and a variety of abnormal, physiological processes throughout the brain may combine to produce a clinical syndrome in its fullest manifestation. Furthermore, the contributions of potential underlying mechanisms may be different for different patients with MIND due to different etiologies (i.e., blunt-force trauma versus blast-exposure versus severe febrile illness in adulthood).

Kindling Model

Kindling of neural circuitry is a physiological method for producing seizures in lower species of animals, a laboratory process that was first described in 1969 (Goddard, 1969). The process of kindling (and its cousins, "partial kindling" and "sensitization") have been invoked as an experimental model for human psychiatric and behavior disorders ranging from bipolar disorder to anxiety disorders and from PTSD to personality change in epilepsy. This frequent invoking of kindling as an explanatory construct led one expert on kindling to title an article: "Does kindling model anything relevant?" (Adamec, 1990).

In addition to being invoked to account for too many different types of psychiatric disorders, a major weakness of any kindling model of human psychopathology is that kindling has never been definitively demonstrated to occur in human beings. There are two basic reasons for this state of affairs. First, it would be unethical to try to "kindle" epileptic seizures in a human being because man generally is not regarded as an experimental animal for such invasive procedures. Hence, the relevant studies cannot be performed ethically. Second, animal research has demonstrated that it apparently becomes increasingly difficult to produce a full kindling effect in more highly evolved species with a greater degree of encephalization (Neppe & Tucker, 1988). Thus, kindling remains at present a provocative model for the development of abnormal electrical activity in the human brain.

Basically, kindling involves the periodic application of an initially subconvulsive electrical or chemical stimulus to brain tissue. At first application, subthreshold stimulation fails to evoke a clinical seizure or any EEG abnormality; however, with repeated applications, the same stimulus eventually will produce changes in ongoing animal behavior, EEG changes, and eventually generalized seizures with clonic muscle contractions (Pollock, 1985). After an animal's brain has been "kindled," each subsequent application of the electrical or chemical stimulus will progress to a full motor seizure; after a brain has been kindled, spontaneous seizures and abnormal inter-ictal discharges on EEG also may be observed. Kindling is fairly easy to produce in rats and cats, but more difficult to produce in more highly evolved primates (Wada, Mizoguchi, & Komai, 1985; Wada & Tsuchimochi, 1995).

Different areas of the brain exhibit considerable variation in the threshold of stimulation necessary to kindle a seizure disorder. The gray matter of the cerebral neocortex is far more resistant to kindling than are limbic structures such as the amygdala, olfactory bulb, the pyriform cortex, and hippocampus (Burnham, 2002; Pollock, 1985). Furthermore, stimulus thresholds for kindling are not only low in limbic structures, but they tend to drop even lower with repeated stimulation (Burnham, 2002).

The term "kindling" makes reference to starting a fire. A small amount of kindling, if carefully ignited, can result in a larger fire, one that can ignite a larger pile of wood, or even an entire forest. When explaining the concept of kindling to lay people, we also sometimes use the analogy of recruitment. A small number of kindled cells in a vulnerable area appear to be able to recruit other neurons to develop abnormal electrical activity, so that, eventually, a fairly sizeable pool of neurons all will fire synchronously. When enough cells fire together (i.e., when enough cells in a certain area of the brain have been recruited), changes in ongoing behavior will be manifest, followed by EEG changes on the surface on the brain. The eventual involvement of the motor system and the rest of the brain then will produce a conventional generalized seizure.

"Partial kindling" refers to the process of repeatedly stimulating the brain, but only to the point where subthreshold stimulation produces intermediate behavioral changes in an animal —changes that do not then progress to become full-blown motor seizures (Adamec, 2001). Thus, a partially kindled cat may assume a defensive posture following electrical stimulation but not progress to manifest frank motor seizures. Observations on partially kindled animals suggest that ongoing human behavior also might be disrupted by subclinical electrical discharges in the brain that are nevertheless insufficient to produce conventional epileptic seizures in man.

A "whiplash" model of brain injury developed by Liu has demonstrated gradual EEG changes in the hippocampi of rhesus monkeys, a process that seems quite compatible with the time-course that would be consistent with a partial kindling process in human beings (Liu, Chandran, Heath, & Unterharnscheidt, 1984).This model also is consistent with acceleration-deceleration brain injury producing symptoms of MIND following traffic accidents (Mamelak, 2000). Unfortunately, it appears that no subsequent work was published by these authors employing this potentially heuristic model of acceleration-deceleration injury.

If future research were to establish a better-defined role for kindling or partial kindling in the development of MIND, then, theoretically, attention could be focused on preventing or mitigating such processes pharmacologically with antikindling medications in the acute phase of the injury to eliminate or reduce the spread of neuro-electric dysfunction in the post-acute period.

Deafferentation Model

Deafferentation means eliminating or reducing nerve impulses that project to a particular region of the brain by cutting afferent neurons. (Afferent neurons are those whose axons connect to the dendrites of other neurons.) With experimental animals, this often is accomplished by undercutting the grey matter of the cerebral cortex to eliminate input from underlying white matter fiber tracts that lie beneath cortical grey matter. When normal input to an area of cortical neurons was eliminated by such undercutting in cats, paroxysmal brain wave activity began in 40% of the animals within 2–3 hours in the area of the cortex immediately adjacent to the cortex that was undercut (Topolnik, Steriade, & Timofeev, 2003). In the authors words,

> The seizures that followed the undercut consisted of spike-wave/polyspike complexes and fast runs, resembling the electrographic patterns of some clinical epileptic syndromes. An increased local synchrony in the relatively intact cortex evolved into paroxysmal activity that ultimately spread to the deafferented cortex. . . . These results indicated that alterations in neuronal synchrony following neuronal trauma can be a critical factor in triggering electrographic seizures." (p. 883)

Thus, depriving a small area of the cerebral cortex of its customary afferent input produced a state of hyper-excitability in the *adjacent* cortex with EEG evidence of seizure-like electrical abnormalities.

Research from other laboratories has produced similar findings in rats (Graber & Prince, 2004; Prince et al., 2009). Using a rat undercutting model of the development of epilepsy, Graber & Prince (2004) further demonstrated that there was a "critical period" of time for the prevention of cortical hyper-excitability:

> We propose that the hyperexcitability caused by partial cortical isolation may represent an early stage of post-

traumatic epileptogenesis. A hypothetical cascade of events leading to subsequent pathophysiological activity is likely initiated at the time of injury but remains plastic during this critical period. (p. 86)

This suggests the possibility that pharmacological intervention in the acute stage of injury might diminish the potential for seizure development later. In addition to creating neuronal hyper-excitability, undercutting also is likely to produce a second pathological process, one that leads to defects in GABAnergic neuronal transmission and reduced inhibitory control of neuronal firing (Prince et al., 2009). This is of interest because most anticonvulsants act to increase the inhibitory role of the neurotransmitter GABA in the brain.

Clearly, mild-to-moderate TBI in human beings does not produce such precise and thorough undercutting of white matter input to the human cortex. However, damage to white matter following blunt-force trauma following even mild TBI is a well-documented phenomenon (Kraus et al., 2007; Niogi et al., 2008; Scheid, Walther, Guthke, Preul, & von Cramon, 2006; Wozniak et al., 2007). Diffuse axonal injury is observed frequently due to neuronal shearing and stretching and to rotational forces, rather than the sort of artificial undercutting used in animal research on epilepsy. However, if the extent of blunt-force trauma were sufficient to partially "disconnect" white matter axons from reaching grey matter dendrites in adequate numbers, then a similar state of neuronal hyper-excitability might lead to the development of seizure-like symptoms in human patients. In fact, a recent study that combined both structural neuro-imaging (i.e., MRI with DTI) and cognitive testing strongly suggested that such partial disconnection does occur between the thalamus (a major sensory relay station) and portions of the human cortex following even mild TBI (Little et al., 2010). The authors further speculated that this type of diffuse axonal injury may have an adverse effect of cognitive functioning. Although admittedly speculative, such a proposition is consistent with the observation that the extent of axonal damage to white matter fibers is a key predictor of functional outcome in a wide variety of neuro-pathological processes in human beings (Medana & Esiri, 2003).

Additional support for the potential relevance of the deaf-ferentation process to outcome in mild TBI was found in the multimodal imaging study recently conducted by Huang and colleagues (2009). These investigators used MRI scans with DTI to document damage to white matter fiber tracts and magneto-encephalography (MEG) to study abnormal slow-wave activity from the cortex in patients with mild TBI who continued to experience symptoms of Persistent Post-Concussive Syndrome. The slow waves coming from the cortices of the mild TBI patients originated from areas of cortical gray matter that had experienced deafferentation due to axonal injuries in underlying white matter, as demonstrated on MRI with DTI. This was true for patients with mild TBI following blunt-force trauma and for patients with mild TBI following blast exposure. In the words of the authors:

> In the present study, we showed that our integrated imaging approach with MEG slow wave imaging and DTI measurements can detect subtle neuronal injuries that are not visible using conventional neuroimaging methods (e.g., CT and MRI). Furthermore, our results showed that axonal injury in patients with mild TBI caused the co-occurrence of abnormal MEG slow waves in cortical gray matter areas and abnormally reduced anisotropy in white matter fiber tracts. Specifically, for the first time in humans, we showed that abnormal MEG slow waves accrued from cortical gray matter neurons that connect to white matter fibers with axonal injury, and axonal injury due to tissue shearing and stretching also led to reduction of anisotropy in white matter tracts, which was detected by DTI. These results are consistent with the previous animal studies in cats . . . and support our hypothesis that the pathological cortical gray matter de-afferentation detected by MEG is directly related to the axonal injury as measured by DTI in the white matter

fibers that connect with the slow wave generating gray matter areas. (p. 1221)

Furthermore, the authors concluded that the " . . . existence of abnormal MEG slow waves in all 10 mild TBI patients was consistent with the persistence of their post-concussive symptoms" (p. 1224). In addition, other research suggests that it may be the total amount of cortical deafferentation throughout the brain that determines whether focal hyper-excitability of the cortex results in abnormal cortical activity in any single locus that has been deprived of normal white matter input (Frohlich, Bazhenov, & Sejnowski, 2008). Although Huang's research team did not specifically interview for MIND-like symptoms, their findings suggest that deafferentation models of traditional epilepsy may have relevance for the development of focal electrical abnormalities, which may be associated with episodic symptoms following mild TBI.

Hippocampal Model

The structures included in the hippocampal complex on the mesial aspects of both temporal lobes have a crucial role in processing sensory input into a coherent form that permits later retrieval or episodic memories from long-term memory storage. It is one of the sites where multiple, sensory inputs converge in the brain, and this region has strong connections with the amygdala deeper in the temporal lobe, a crucial area involved in mediating the emotions of fear and anger. Furthermore, the hippocampus and adjacent structures are especially vulnerable to damage from both trauma and hypoxia and fairly easily kindled in subhuman species. Gouvier and his colleagues (Ryan et al., 2006) have provided a succinct summary of the model, which initially was articulated by Hines (Hines, Swan, Roberts, & Varney, 1995).

Hines, Swan, Roberts, and Varney (1995) suggested a neurophysiological model that explains how a relatively small amount of damage to critical inhibitory cells within the

> hippocampus may result in the presentation of multiple, partial seizure-like symptoms. Specifically, these investigators hypothesize that the excitatory output of the hippocampus is increased following the loss of inhibitory influence of granule cells in the dentate, secondary to head injury. (p. 290)

One of the attractive features of this model is that it can explain how damage to a relatively small group of neurons in a crucial location could result in the development of so many intermittent psycho-sensory, cognitive, and affective symptoms. However, no autopsy studies on MIND-like patients have yet been published; nor, to our knowledge, have any fine-grained studies of the dentate gyrus using MRI with DTI following mild TBI—the sort of evidence that would be needed to provide definitive support for this "hippocampal" model.

Since this model first was proposed roughly 15 years ago, it also has been established that the human brain has the capacity to produce new neurons well into adulthood. Thus, it is also possible that the death of cells in and around the hippocampal complex could trigger the growth of new cells (i.e., neurogenesis) that also could influence the inhibitory/excitatory balance of hippocampal output (Balu & Lucki, 2009). However, it is presently unclear whether such neurogenesis results in improved brain function or disrupted brain function. As one expert has remarked,

> New synapses are aberrant, since they are formed in regions in which they are not present in controls. They also involved receptors that are not present in controls, and this facilitates the generation of seizures. Therefore, an aberrant form of reactive neuronal plasticity provides a substrate for the long-lasting sequelae of seizures. Since these events take place in brain structures involved in the integrative and mnemonic [i.e., memory] functions, they will have an important impact. (Ben-Ari, 2008, p. 17)

Ben-Ari's skepticism regarding beneficial versus harmful effects of spontaneous neural regeneration was consistent with the conclusions drawn by Sutula & Dudek (2007):

The recognition that mossy fiber sprouting [in the dentate gyrus] is induced after hippocampal injury and seizures and contributes conditionally to the emergence of recurrent excitation has provided a conceptual framework for understanding how injury and seizure-induced reorganization may contribute to paroxysmal network synchronization, epileptogenesis, and the consequences of repeated seizures, and thus has had a major influence on fundamental aspect of the epilepsies. (p. 541)

Similar conclusions also have been published by Parent (2007) and Kaneko & Sawamoto (2009).

At any rate, what does seem clear is that the dentate gyrus and hippocampal region are sites of much continuing interest in research on the development of conventional epilepsy (Blumcke et al., 2009; Hunt, Scheff, & Smith, 2009; Morgan & Soltesz, 2008; Seress et al., 2009; Zhang & Buckmaster, 2009).

Pre-ictal (or Prodromal) Changes in Brain Physiology Prior to Seizure Onset

Among others, epileptologist Ernst Niedermeyer (2002) has called attention to increased interest in studying the physiology of brain processes, which occur just *prior* to initiation of traditional complex partial seizures (i.e., so-called "temporal lobe epilepsy" or psychomotor seizures—a focal form of epilepsy). He has used the term "pre-aura" for designation of earliest pre-ictal manifestations signaling that a conventional focal seizure will occur in the future. (Ictus means "event" in Latin—in this case: seizure onset; thus, the term "pre-ictal" refers to events occurring immediately prior to seizure onset.) Both early electrical and vascular changes may precede an actual seizure by 1 to 20 minutes, according to Niedermeyer. The typical, clinical course of a traditionally diagnosed, complex partial seizure episode consists of several identifiable stages. The "aura" (Latin for "warning") represents the earliest manifestation of the seizure event (or "ictus"). The episode then progresses, usually in a fairly predictable pattern to motor automatism (e.g., lip-smacking, head turning, aimless movements) and loss of conscious processing of one's surroundings. The post-ictal period may be characterized by some degree of confusion and mental fatigue. (The inter-ictal period refers to the time between the occurrence of discrete seizures.)

According to epileptologist Ernst Niedermeyer, the " . . . pre-aura constitutes a pre-epileptic period in which both EEG and patient behavior [may] fail to indicate an imminent seizure, while the perifocal microcirculation is altered" (p. 58). Thus, extremely small changes in the focal circulation in seizure-producing areas of the brain precede the observable electrical discharges on EEG (i.e., those that constitute the seizure itself). Several groups of researchers have demonstrated pre-aura reductions in micro-focal cerebral blood flow to the areas involved with seizure propagation (e.g., Le Van Quyen, Martinerie, Navarro, Baulac, & Varela, 2001). From case studies, it also seems clear that marked alterations in cognition, emotion, and sensory processing can take place during such a pre-ictal period prior to seizure onset (Shukla et al., 2008).

Research from a team of French epileptologists has demonstrated that there is a period of marked "desynchrony" of brain activity between structures in the frontal and temporal lobes just prior to the onset of marked increase in the synchrony of neuronal firing between these structures that is characteristic of a conventional complex partial seizure (Bartolomei et al., 2005):

> We found that these intense emotional alterations were associated with a decrease of synchrony between signals recorded from neural networks known to be involved in emotional processing, and in particular a loss of synchrony between the orbito-frontal cortex and the amygdala. This disruption of functional connections could then result in the disruption of emotional regulation leading to the release of the altered behavior, as observed in epileptic patients during seizures. . . . We propose that the occurrence of intense ictal emotional behavior disturbance is

related to a disruption of the normal mechanisms of emotional regulation. (p. 2473)

One may, therefore, ask, "What if the micro-reductions in local blood flow and changes in synchrony of brain electrical activity were to persist for a brief period of time but then *failed* to progress to the manifestation of a conventional complex partial seizure episode?" It could be the case that local desynchrony between key brain structures, as demonstrated by Bartolomei and associates (2005) might be sufficient to facilitate transiently disrupted cognition, alterations in emotional tone, and transitory deficits in processing of sensory data consistent with various symptoms of MIND.

Although such a theory has not been previously proposed, it seems clear that subtle (but very real) physiological changes may occur prior to formal seizure-onset. Previous research has documented that inter-ictal spiking (i.e., abnormal electrical activity between seizure episodes) is associated with hypo-metabolism on SPECT scans from the same regions that manifest the spiking (Guillon et al., 1998). It may well be that altered metabolic activity may prove to be a bio-marker for reduced (or otherwise abnormal) function in some focal region(s) of the brain. If such reduced function decreased the firing of key inhibitory neurons, then disruptions in normal brain activity could occur as reversible release phenomena (i.e., transient loss of inhibitory input). Put another way, some MIND-like symptoms could be associated with the equivalent of a focal pre-ictal state, but one which does *not* then progress to the state of increased blood flow seen immediately prior to seizure-onset (Federico, Abbott, Briellmann, Harvey, & Jackson, 2005).

In support of the pre-ictal state or prodromal hypothesis regarding the causation of MIND, Scaramelli and colleagues (Scaramelli et al., 2009) found that prodromal symptoms were reported in 39 out of 100 patients with traditional forms of epilepsy. The most frequent prodromal symptoms were behavioral, cognitive, and mood changes "within the neuropsychiatric domain." When consciously detected, the prodromal changes in their patients often were perceived as gradual in onset (rather than being abrupt) or having a clearly demarcated offset. These investigators concluded:

> The subtle nature of these symptoms, in contrast to other more overt clinical phenomena like motor manifestations, could explain why recognition of prodromes has not been so easy, and why research in this area has not been more extensive in the past. (p. 249)

Interim Summary

A clear etiology for the clinical presentation of MIND remains to be demonstrated. We have presented four speculative models of the possible processes that could relate to etiology of MIND-like symptoms. It is conceivable that elements of these putative models may overlap somewhat or combine to produce the complex clinical picture associated with the episodic symptoms or MIND (i.e., the models are not necessarily mutually exclusive). However, future advances in basic brain science and research on epilepsy are likely to provide important pieces of the puzzle, assuming that a sufficient number of neuroscientists and clinicians come to recognize the existence of MIND as a diagnosable and treatable condition in its own right—a subtype of post-concussive disorder that may well be related to, but separate from, well-established agreed-upon forms of traditional epilepsy.

Are There Any Nonpharmacological or Behavioral Treatments for Treating the Symptoms of MIND?

Some patients express a preference for avoiding prescription medications if at all possible. Among the American public at large, the quests for alternative therapies and holistic healing most likely reflect dissatisfaction with various aspects of the practice of Western medicine in this fast-paced epoch of human history. Such an anti-medication bias appears to have several sources: (1) high costs associated with prescription medications; (2) backlash toward the use of drugs in general as a result of the widespread use of illicit substances; (3) a given patient's perception that he or she is "already taking too many pills"; and (4) concerns about career advancement (e.g., fitness for military duty, truck-driving as a profession, not wishing to be stigmatized as a neuropsychiatric patient).

Unfortunately, as far as we know, currently no effective treatment exists for MIND-like symptoms following blunt-force head trauma that does not involve the regular use of anticonvulsant mood stabilizers, such as valproic acid and carbamazepine (often in conjunction with other types of medication, such as SSRI antidepressants, or additional medication for persistent headaches). This does not necessarily mean that eventually a nonpharmacological treatment might not be developed; however, at the present time, we are simply not aware of any such treatment. Eventually, biofeedback of brain-wave activity using sophisticated, quantitative EEG patterns may have promise for assisting in the rehabilitation of patients following brain injury, but this is not a widespread practice at the present time.

After Optimally Treatment With Medication, How Long Do Patients Need to Continue on a Mood Stabilizer?

The answer is, "We do not know for sure," because we once again lack relevant research data. Only one case (Neppe & Kaplan, 1988) has been published in which a patient with new-onset, MIND-like symptoms was treated effectively for a short period of time and then discontinued taking medication with no subsequent return of symptoms. The clinical observations of the first author on adult patients who have been struggling with chronic, undiagnosed symptoms of MIND for months or years suggest that discontinuing a mood stabilizer (after a successful treatment response has been established) usually results in the return of

MIND-like symptoms. On the other hand, the second author (working clinically in conjunction with Dr. George Phillips) has observed pediatric cases in which the treating physician has successfully tapered patients from carbamazepine without resumption of symptoms. This appears more likely to be possible when treatment has been initiated *soon* after the onset of MIND following an instance of sports concussion. These observations, although unsystematic, suggest that prompt treatment following the acute onset of MIND-like symptoms in younger patients may obviate the need for extended treatment over the course of years. However, more data clearly are needed on this important clinical topic.

At the risk of being repetitive, we want to reiterate that older adolescent and young adult MIND patients often forget or discount how awful they felt prior to successful treatment and are be tempted to wean themselves off of their medications without first consulting their treating physicians. *This virtually always represents a serious mistake in judgment,* and sometimes it can be difficult to re-establish the previous level of good treatment response after two or three such episodes (for reasons that are unclear at this time).Therefore, if you are a treated patient who is reading this book, please *do not make any alterations in your treatment regimen* without consulting your prescribing physician or care provider.

When a Combat Veteran (or Victim of Civilian Assault With Head Trauma) Has Both PTSD From Combat and Persistent Post-Concussive Disorder With MIND-like Symptoms From Blunt-Force Trauma or Blast Exposure, Which Symptoms Should Be Treated First?

Logically, at least four strategies or approaches can be taken to the timing of treatment in such instances: (1) treating PTSD first and then MIND-like symptoms; (2) treating the Persistent Post-Concussive Disorder with MIND-like symptoms first and then the PTSD; (3) treating symptoms from both disorders simultaneously; or (4) treating the symptoms that appear to be causing the patient the greatest distress after an initial assessment has been performed. Of these three options, option (3) would seem to be the least desirable because making two or three therapeutic interventions at once does not permit the prescribing care provider to determine which positive changes were due to which interventions.

In the experience of the first author, most care providers he has observed elect to treat the symptoms of PTSD first. There are several reasons for this preference:

- There are more published "guidelines" and clinical protocols for treating PTSD than there are for treating Persistent Post-Concussive Disorder;

- Many clinicians are not aware of the concept of MIND or, if they are aware, do not think that multiple, episodic symptoms are necessarily associated with "real" neurobehavioral dysfunction;

- Many prescribers feel more comfortable with the use of antidepressant medications (usually the first line of pharmacological treatment of symptoms of PTSD) than they are using mood stabilizers with anticonvulsant properties;

- SSRI antidepressants have relatively fewer serious potential side-effects compared with some of the more serious potential side-effects of anticonvulsant mood-stabilizers;

- There currently are more behavioral or psychotherapeutic options for treating the symptoms of PTSD than for addressing PPCS;

- Early survey studies in populations at increased risk for both PTSD and mild TBI have suggested that physical symptoms may be more strongly associated with PTSD than with TBI (e.g., Hoge et al., 2008).

Thus, in our experience, it is the rare clinician who recognizes and decides to treat the symptoms of Persistent Post-Concussive Disorder with MIND prior to attempting to treat symptoms of comorbid PTSD.

However, a rational argument also can be made for treating the symptoms of MIND first (if they are recognized) and then treating PTSD symptoms second, after optimal management of MIND-like symptoms has been established. First, the vast majority of patients with MIND have memory gaps and cognitive lapses that make it difficult for them to benefit from behavioral or psychotherapeutic interventions for PTSD. After their intermittent cognitive symptoms are treated optimally with an anticonvulsant mood stabilizer, such patients become more amenable to behavioral and emotional interventions (Jonas, 1965). Although excessive anger can be associated with both MIND and PTSD, mood stabilizers help to decrease angry outbursts due to subclinical electrophysiological dysfunction, and this is of direct benefit to family dynamics and job adjustment because episodes of unpredictable rage are among the most aversive symptoms of MIND for family, friends, and co-workers of patients with MIND. Because behavioral treatment for combat-related PTSD generally involves some type of exposure to distressing memories of traumatic events, it makes sense to have achieved an optimal level of brain function pharmacologically before the patient tackles this portion of PTSD treatment. To put it another way: What sense does it make to induce even greater emotional stress in an already physiologically dysfunctional and stressed brain?

Ruff, however, makes a cogent case for focusing on treating the most distressing symptoms, particularly when they are commonly treatable symptoms such as headache, poor sleep, and chronic pain from other medical conditions (Ruff, Ruff, & Wang, 2008). This approach also makes a certain amount of sense and lays the foundation for a strong partnership between patient and care provider if progress in these areas can be achieved quickly. Additional considerations for treating combat veterans with mild TBI and PTSD are presented in the recently issued "VA/DoD

Clinical Practice Guideline for Management of Concussion/Mild Traumatic Brain Injury" (Management of Concussion/mTBI Working Group, 2009).

Is There Currently a Single Diagnostic Test That Is Specific for MIND?

Unfortunately, the answer to this question is "No." Some investigators have suggested that injection of the pro-convulsant drug procaine is likely to provoke MIND-like symptoms in patients with dysfunction in the limbic regions of their brains (e.g., Pollock, 1985; Servan-Schreiber, Perlstein, Cohen, & Mintum, 1998). Injection with procaine appears to promote the experiencing of multiple, intermittent symptoms in vulnerable individuals and, thus, theoretically could be of some value in providing evidence of excessive excitability of limbic system structures. However, use of this protocol can be subjectively quite unpleasant, and it has never been fully developed as an accepted neuropsychiatric test procedure.

Functional neuro-imaging studies such as SPECT scans (Stinson, 2001) have been found to be useful in documenting areas of reduced blood flow in the brain even when CT and MRI scans for structural damage have been negative following blunt-force trauma. However, it appears that other clinical conditions besides head trauma are associated with decreased areas of perfusion in the anterior portions of the brain. This means that, although SPECT scans may prove to be highly *sensitive* to cerebral dysfunction following brain trauma, they may not be *specific* in identifying the effects of such trauma. Still, in a controversial area such as diagnosis of mild TBI, obtained measures of brain *function*, such as SPECT or PET scans, can provide some measure of corroboration when there are interview data and neuro-cognitive test findings (e.g., marked dichotic listening impairment in the absence of a structural lesion) suggestive of PPCS with MIND-like symptoms.

MRI scans with diffuse tensor tractography may identify minute changes associated with structural damage to the brain, even when the results of standard CT and MRI scans have been negative (Lipton et al., 2008). The combined use of MRI with DTI and magnetoencephalography has been used to demonstrate deafferentation (i.e., separation between subcortical white matter and cortical gray matter) in patients with persistent Post-Concussive Disorder following mild TBI (Huang et al. 2009). However, currently roughly 20 facilities in North America have the capability to perform magneto-encephalography, and these tend to be in heavily populated, urban areas. This relative lack of diagnostic resources suggests that magneto-encephalography will not become a routinely available diagnostic test in the near future.

Trudeau et al. (1998) found that quantitative EEG (qEEG) could be used to differentiate patients with long-term PTSD from patients with long-term PTSD plus blast exposure in combat. However, no similar studies have been published with quantitative EEG with blast-exposed veterans from Iraq and Afghanistan. Curiously, the Trudeau study is seldom-cited in current reviews of shell-shock and mild TBI, perhaps because it was accomplished following the Vietnam War and Desert Storm but prior to the Global War on Terror.

The neuropsychological test that is most frequently failed by patients with MIND-like symptoms following blunt-force trauma appears to be Dichotic Word Listening (Meyers, Roberts, Bayless, Volkert, & Evitts, 2002; Richardson, Springer, Varney, Struchen, & Roberts, 1994). However, replication of these findings has not been accomplished yet in blunt-force trauma or blast-exposed patients from the OIF/OEF conflicts.

Ruff, Ruff, and Wang (2008) demonstrated that reduced sense of smell was the single most common finding in blast-exposed patients with persistent headaches. However, reduced sense of smell also can be caused by a variety of factors. Furthermore, many care providers (e.g., neurologists, psychologists, and clinical neuropsychologists) defer testing olfaction for reasons that are not always documented. Given Ruff's findings (2008) and recent research by Fortin et al. (Fortin, Lefebvre, & Ptito, 2010) regarding the frequency of olfactory impairment following mild

TBI, such cross-disciplinary reluctance to formally test olfaction may prove to be a regrettable oversight clinically.

In summary, the diagnosis of MIND presently relies largely upon interview data supported by findings from multiple neuro-diagnostic modalities. Hopefully, this state of affairs eventually will change with additional research.

When a Patient Produces a High Score on the Iowa Interview, Does This *Always* Signify That the Patient Is Suffering From MIND Due to Some Sort of Physical Brain Trauma?

Not necessarily. Some highly dissociative patients, such as those with Dissociative Identity Disorder (i.e., what used to be referred to as Multiple Personality Disorder) or severe PTSD with ego-state pathology may produce high scores on the Iowa Interview due to excessive use of the process of dissociation (Bob, Glaslova, Susta, Jasova, & Raboch, 2006; Bob, Sista, Pavlat, Hynek, & Raboch, 2005; Ross, 1994). Due to abrupt shifts in conscious awareness (rather than subclinical electrophysiological dysfunction), dissociative individuals may report fleeting sensory symptoms, disrupted cognition, and brief mood swings (which some clinicians believe may represent partial trauma memories divorced from full recall of the entire traumatic incident associated with the specific mood).

With specific regard to the Iowa Interview, Roca & Freeman (2002) administered a questionnaire form of the Iowa Interview to patients with combat-related PTSD and normal comparison subjects. They found that the PTSD group endorsed significantly more intermittent symptoms than did controls. However, these investigators did not rule out possible confounding effects of head injury; blast exposure; medication regimens; effects of severe febrile illness in adulthood; or comorbid nonsubstance-abuse psychiatric diagnoses. Thus, it is difficult to know exactly what to make of their results. They had been hoping to demonstrate a rationale for the use of anticonvulsant mood stabilizers in patients with chronic PTSD (i.e., based on elevated number of intermittent symptoms). However, the most recent data indicate that treatment with valproic acid has few, if any, positive effects on symptoms of chronic PTSD (Davis et al., 2008; Hamner et al., 2009).

Wong, Regenitter, and Barrios (1994) studied the vulnerability of a questionnaire version of the Iowa Interview to exaggerated or feigned responding by using different instructional sets. Students who were instructed to simulate the effects of head injury reported more symptoms on the Iowa Interview than normal comparison subjects who had not been so instructed. However, mean total score of the simulator group did not begin to approach the mean scores produced by clinical samples of actual MIND patients. Thus, even when instructed to respond in an exaggerated fashion, the average response of young adults simulating head injury was well within the normal range. Although it surely is not impossible to fake bad on the Iowa Interview (or any interview, for that matter), outright lying or feigning of symptoms does not seem to be a common occurrence in our clinical experiences. Roberts et al. (1992) tested a version of the Iowa Interview with six improbable foil questions, only to find that real patients almost never endorsed the bogus items. Thus, the six foil items were omitted from subsequent versions of the Iowa Interview (Roberts, 1999).

After Symptoms of MIND Are Optimally Treated, Does That Result in Full Functional Recovery?

Not necessarily, unfortunately. Other permanent deficits still may interfere with job performance, educational performance, or social functioning. This is especially true when numerous intermittent symptoms had the effects of masking the full extent of difficulties with executive function (Wozniak et al., 2007) prior to successful treatment of MIND-like symptoms. In the words of Verduyn and colleagues (Verduyn et al. 1992), " . . . reduction in the frequency and severity of episodic, partial seizure-like symptoms did not always guarantee a return to full functional status; this was particularly true for patients who manifested clear evidence of frontal lobe dysfunction on neuropsychological evaluation or family interview" (p. 254–255). Executive function refers to a person's capacity to manage their lives in a coherent, self-regulated, and planned fashion; to organize their thoughts and behavior to meet the demands of social situations; to make effective decisions; to prioritize tasks; and to manage their time efficiently. Deficits in executive function most often are associated with damage to the prefrontal region of the brain and can pose difficult challenges for neuro-rehabilitation. Damage to the prefrontal regions is most likely to occur following instances of mild TBI with frontal and occipital impact.

References

Adamec, R. E. (1990). Does kindling model anything clinically relevant? *Biological Psychiatry, 27,* 249–279.

Adamec, R. E. (2001). Partial kindling and behavioral pathologies. *International Review of Neurobiology, 45,* 409–434.

Agrawal, A., Timothy, J., Pandit, L., & Maniu, M. (2006). Post-traumatic epilepsy: An overview. *Clinical Neurology and Neurosurgery, 108,* 433–439.

Balu, D. T., & Lucki, I. (2009). Adult hippocampal neurogenesis: Regulation, functional implications, and contribution to disease pathology. *Neuroscience and Biobehavioral Research, 33,* 232–252.

Ben-Ari, Y. (2008). Epilepsies and neuronal plasticity: For better or for worse? *Dialogues in Clinical Neuroscience, 10,* 17–27.

Blumcke, I., Vinters, H. V., Armstrong, D., Aronica, E., Thom, M., & Spreafico, R., (2009). Malformations of cortical development and epilepsies: Neuropathological findings with emphasis on focal cortical dysplasia. *Epileptic Disorders, 11,* 181–193.

Bob, P., Glaslova, K., Susta, M., Jasova, D., & Raboch, J. (2006). Traumatic dissociation, epileptic-like phenomena, and schizophrenia. *Neurology and Endocrinology Letters, 27,* 321–326.

Bob, P., Susta, M., Paylat, J., Hynek, K., & Raboch, J. (2005). Depression, traumatic dissociation and epileptic-like phenomena. *Neurology and Endocrinology Letters, 26*, 321–325.

Bridgers, S. L. (1988). Ambulatory cassette electroencephalography of psychiatric patients. *Archives of Neurology, 45*, 71–74.

Burnham, W. M. (2002). Why are complex partial seizures intractable? *Advances in Experimental Medicine and Biology, 497*, 107–110.

Davis, L. L., Davison, J. R., Ward, L. C., Bartolucci, A., Bowden, C. L., & Petty, F. (2008). Divalproex in the treatment of posttraumatic stress disorder: A randomized, double-blind, placebo-controlled trial in an veteran population. *Journal of Clinical Psychopharmacology, 28*, 84–88.

Federico, P., Abbott, D. F., Briellman, R. S., Harvey, A. S., & Jackson, G. D. (2005). Functional MRI of the pre-ictal state. *Brain, 128*, 1811–1817.

Fortin, A., Lefebvre, M. B., & Ptito, M. (2010). Traumatic brain injury and olfactory deficits: the tale of two smell tests! *Brain Injury, 24*, 27–33.

Frohlich, F., Bazhenov, M., & Sejnowski, T.J. (2008). Pathological effect of homeostatic synaptic scaling on network dynamics in disease of the cortex. *Journal of Neuroscience, 28*, 1709–1720.

Goddard, G. V., McIntyre, D. C., & Leech, C. K. (1969). A permanent change in brain function resulting from daily electrical stimulation. *Experimental Neurology, 25*, 295–330.

Grote, C. L., Pierre-Louis, S. J., Smith, M. C., Roberts, R. J., & Varney, N. R. (1995). Significance of unilateral ear extinction on the dichotic listening test. *Journal of Clinical and Experimental Neuropsychology, 17*, 1–8.

Graber, K. D., & Prince, D. A. (2004). A critical period for prevention of posttraumatic neocortical hyperexcitability in rats. *Annals of Neurology, 55*, 860–970.

Guillon, B., Duncan, R., Biraben, A., Bernard, A. M., Vignal, J. P., & Chauvel, P. Correlation between interictal regional cerebral blood flow and depth-recorded interictal spiking in temporal lobe epilepsy. *Epilepsia, 39*, 67–76.

Hamner, M. B., Faldowski, R. A., Robert, S., Ulmer, H. G., Horner, M. D., & Lorberbaum, J. P. (2009). A preliminary controlled trial of divalproex in posttraumatic stress disorder. *Annals of Clinical Psychiatry, 21*, 89–94.

Heath, C., & Heath, D. (2007). *Made to stick.* New York, NY: Random House.

Hines, M., Swan, C., Roberts, R. J., & Varney, N. R. (1995). Characteristics and mechanisms of epilepsy spectrum disorder: An explanatory model. *Applied Neuropsychology, 2*, 1–6.

Hoge, C. W., McGurk, D., Thomas, J. L., Cox, A. L., Engel, C. C., & Castro, C. A. (2008). Mild traumatic brain injury in U.S. Soldiers returning from Iraq. *New England Journal of Medicine, 358*, 453–463.

Huang, M., Theilman, R. J., Robb, A., Angeles, A., Nichols, S., Drake, A., . . . Lee, R. R. (2009). Integrating imaging approach with MEG and DTI to detect mild traumatic brain injury in military and civilian patients. *Journal of Neurotrauma*, Epub ahead of publication.

Hunt, R. F., Scheff, S. W., & Smith, B. N. (2009). Posttraumatic epilepsy after controlled cortical impact injury in mice. *Experimental Neurology*, 215, 243–252.

Hutt, S. J. (1972). Experimental analysis of brain activity and behavior in children with "minor" seizures. *Epilepsia, 13*, 520–534.

Jonas, A. D. (1965). *Ictal and subictal neurosis.* Springfield, IL.: C.C. Thomas.

Jorge, R. E., & Starkstein, S. E. (2005). Pathophysiological aspects of major depression following traumatic brain injury. *Journal of Head Trauma Rehabilitation, 20*, 475–487.

Kaneko, N., & Sawamoto, K. (2009). Adult neurogenesis and its alteration under pathological conditions. *Neuroscience Research, 63*, 155–164.

Kraus, M. F., Susmaras, T., Caughlin, B. P., Walker, C. J., Sweeney, J. A., & Little, D. M. (2007). White matter integrity and cognition in chronic traumatic brain injury: A diffusion tensor imaging study. *Brain, 130*, 2508–2519.

Kutcher, J. S., & Eckner, J. T. (2010). At-risk populations in sports-related concussion. *Current Sports Medicine Reports*, *9*, 16–20.

Lee, G. P., Loring, D. W., Varney, N. R., Roberts, R. J., Newell, J. R., Martin, J. A., . . . Murro, A. M. (1994). Do dichotic word listening asymmetries predict side of temporal lobe seizure onset? *Epilepsy Research*, *19*, 153-160.

Le Van Quyen, M., Martinerie, J., Navarro, V., Baluac, A. M., & Varela, F. J. (2001). Characterizing neurodynamic changes before seizures. *Journal of Clinical Neurophysiology*, *18*, 191–208.

Liu, Y. K., Chandran, K. B., Heath, R. B., & Unterharnscheidt, F. (1984). Subcortical EEG chances in rhesus monkeys following experimental hyper-extension-hyperflexion (whiplash). *Spine*, *9*, 329–338.

Lipton, M. L., Gellella, E., Lo, C., Gold, T., Ardekani, B. A., Shifteh, K., . . . Branch, C. A., (2008). Multifocal white matter ultrastructural abnormalities in mild traumatic brain injury with cognitive disability: A voxel-wise analysis of diffusion tensor imaging. *Journal of Neurotrauma*, *25*, 1335–1342.

Little, D. M., Kraus, M. F., Joseph, J., Geary, E. K., Susmaras, T., Zhou, X. J., . . . Gorelick, P. B. (2010). Thalamic integrity underlines executive dysfunction in traumatic brain injury. *Neurology*, *16*, 558–564.

Loscher W. (2009). Preclinical assessment of proconvulsant drug activity and its relevance for predicting adverse events in humans. *European Journal of Pharmacology*, *21*, 1–11.

Mamelak, M. (2000). The motor vehicle collision injury syndrome. *Neuropsychiatry, Neuropsychology, and Behavioral Neurology*, *13*, 125–135.

Management of Concussion/mTBI Working Group. (2009). VA/DoD clinical practice guideline for management of concussion/mild traumatic brain injury. *Journal of Rehabilitation Research and Development*, *46*, CP1–CP68.

Medana, I. M., & Esiri, M. M. (2003). Axonal damage: A key predictor of outcome in human CNS disease. *Brain*, *126*, 515–530.

Meyers, J. E., Roberts, R. J., Bayless, J. D., Volkert, K., & Evitts, P. E. (2002). Dichotic listening: Expanded norms and clinical application. *Archives of Clinical Neuropsychology*, *17*, 79–90.

Morgan, R. J., & Soltesz, I. (2008). Nonrandom connectivity of the epileptic dentate gyrus predicts a major role for neuronal hubs in seizures. *Processes of the National Academy of Science (USA)*, *105*, 6179–6184.

Niedermeyer, E. (2002). The epileptic pre-aura. *Clinical Electroencephalography*, *33*, 58–61.

Neppe, V. M., & Kaplan, C. (1988). Short-term treatment of atypical spells with carbamazepine. *Clinical Neuropharmacology*, *11*, 287–289.

Neppe, V. N., & Tucker, G. J. (1988). Modern perspective on epilepsy in relation to psychiatry. *Hospital and Community Psychiatry*, *39*. 389–396.

Niogi, S. S., Mukherjee, P., Ghajar, J., Johnson, C., Kolster, R. A., Sarkar, R., . . . McCandliss, B. D. (2008). Extent of microstructural white matter injury in postconcussive syndrome correlates with impaired cognitive reaction time: A 3T diffusion tensor imaging study of mild traumatic brain injury. *American Journal of Neuroradiology*, *29*, 967–973.

Parent, J. M. (2007). Adult neurogenesis in the intact and epileptic dentate gyrus. *Progress in Brain Research*, *163*, 529–540.

Pollock, D. C. (1985). The kindling phenomenon and a clinical application: The procaine test. *Psychiatry Journal of the University of Ottawa*, *10*, 185–192.

Prince, D. A., Parada, I., Scalise, K., Graber, K., Jin, X., & Shen, F. (2009). Epilepsy following cortical injury: Cellular and molecular mechanism as targets for potential prophylaxis. *Epilepsia*, *50*(Suppl. 2), 30–40.

Richardson, E. D., Springer, J. A., Varney, N. R., Struchen, M. A., & Roberts, R. J. (1994). Dichotic listening in the clinic: New neuropsychological applications. *Clinical Neuropsychologist*, *8*, 416–428.

Roberts, R. J. (1999). Epilepsy Spectrum Disorder in the context of mild traumatic brain injury. In N. R. Varney & R. J. Roberts (Eds.), *The evaluation and treatment of mild traumatic brain injury* (pp. 409–447). Mahwah, NJ: Lawrence Erlbaum.

Roberts, R. J., Gorman, L. L., Lee, G. P., Hines, M. E., Richardson, E. D., Riggle, T. A., & Varney, N. R. (1992). The phenomenology of multiple partial seizure-like symptoms without stereotyped spells: An epilepsy spectrum disorder? *Epilepsy Research, 13,* 167–177.

Roberts, R. J., Varney, N. R., Paulsen, J. S., & Richardson, E. D. (1990). Dichotic listening and complex partial seizures. *Journal of Clinical and Experimental Neuropsychology, 12,* 448–458.

Roca, V., & Freeman, T. W. (2002). Psychosensory symptoms in combat veterans with posttraumatic stress disorder. *Journal of Neuropsychiatry and Clinical Neuroscience, 14,* 185–189.

Ross, C. (1994). *The Osiris Complex.* Toronto: University of Toronto Press.

Ruff, R. L., Ruff, S. S., & Wang, X. F. (2008). Headaches among Operation Iraqi Freedom/Operation Enduring Freedom veterans with mild traumatic brain injury associated with exposures to explosions. *Journal of Rehabilitation Research and Development, 45,* 941–952.

Ryan, L. M., O'Jile, J. R., Parks-Levy, J., Betz, B., Hilsabeck, R. C., & Gouvier, W. D. (2006). Complex partial seizure symptom endorsement in individuals with a history of head injury. *Archives of Clinical Neuropsychology, 21,* 287–291.

Scaramelli, A., Braga, P., Avellanal, A., Bogacz, A., Camejo, C., Rega, I., . . . Arciere, B. (2009). Prodromal symptoms in epileptic patients: Clinical characterization of the pre-ictal phase. *Seizure, 18,* 246–250.

Schied, R., Walther, K., Guthke, T., Preul, C., & von Cramon, D. Y. (2006). Cognitive sequelae of diffuse axonal injury. *Archives of Neurology, 63,* 418–424.

Seress, L., Abraham, H., Horvath, Z., Doczi, T., Janszky, J., Klemm, J. . . . Bakay, R. A. (2009). Survival of mossy cells of the hippocampal dentate gyrus in humans with mesial temporal lobe epilepsy. *Journal of Neurosurgery, 111,* 1237–1247.

Servan-Schreiber, D., Perlstein, W. M., Cohen, J. D., & Mintum, M. (1998). Selective pharmacological activation of limbic structures in human volunteers: A positron emission tomography study. *Journal of Neuropsychiatry and Clinical Neuroscience, 10,* 148–159.

Shukla, G., Singh, S., Goyal, V., Gaikwas, S., Srivastaya, A., Bai, C. S., . . . Behari, M. (2008). Prolonged preictal psychosis in refractory seizures: a report of three cases. *Epilepsy and Behavior*, *13*, 252–255.

Statler, K. D., Swank, S., Abildskov, T., Bigler, E. D., & White, H. S. (2008). Traumatic brain injury during developmental reduceds minimal clonic seizure thresholds at maturity. *Epilepsy Research*, *80*, 163–170.

Stinson, G. (2001). "He was never quite himself after that accident": Exploring the long-term consequences of mild traumatic brain injury. *American Journal of Neuroradiology*, *22*, 425–426.

Sutula, T. P., & Dudek, F. E. (2007). Unmasking recurrent excitation by mossy fiber sprouting in the epileptic dentate gyrus: An emergent property of a complex system. *Progress in Brain Research*, *163*, 541–563.

Taylor, M. A. (1999). *Fundamentals of clinical neuropsychiatry*. New York, NY: Oxford University Press.

Topolnik, L., Steriade, M., & Timofeev, I. (2003). Partial cortical deafferentation promotes development of paroxysmal activity. *Cerebral Cortex*, *13*, 883–893.

Trudeau, D. L., Anderson, J., Hansen, L. M., Shagalov, D. N., Schmoller, J., Nugent, S., . . . Barton, S. (1998). Findings of mild traumatic brain injury in combat veterans with PTSD and a history of blast concussion. *Journal of Neuropsychiatry and Clinical Neuroscience*, *10*, 308–313.

Tucker, G. J., Price, T. R. P. Johnson, V. B., & McAllister, T. (1986). Phenomenology of temporal lobe dysfunction: A link to atypical psychosis—a series of cases. *Journal of Nervous and Mental Disease*, *174*, 348–356.

Verduyn, W. H., Hilt, J., Roberts, M. A., & Roberts, R. J. (1992). Multiple partial seizure-like symptoms following "minor" head injury. *Brain Injury*, *6*, 245–260.

Wada, J. A., Mizoguchi, T., & Komai, S. (1985). Kindling epileptogenesis in orbital and mesial frontal cortical areas of subhuman primate. *Epilepsia*, *26*, 472–479.

Wada, J. A., & Tsuchimochi, H. (1995). Cingulate kindling in Senegalese baboons, Papio papio. *Epilepsia*, *36*, 1142–1151.

Wang, C. C., Schoenberg, B. S., Li, S. C., Yang, Y. C., Cheng, X. M., & Bolis, C. L. (1986). Brain injury due to head trauma:

Epidemiology in urban areas of the People's Republic of China. *Archives of Neurology, 43*, 570–572.

Wieser, H. G., Hailermariam, M., Regard, M., & Landis, T. (1992). Unilateral limbic epileptic status activity: Stereo EEG, behavioral, and cognitive data. *Epilepsia, 26*, 19–29.

Wong, J. L., Regenitter, R. P., & Barrios, F. (1994). Base rate and simulated symptoms of mild head injury among normals. *Archives of Clinical Neuropsychology, 9*, 411–425.

Wozniak, J. R., Krach, L., Ward, E., Mueller, B. A., Muetzel, R., Schnoebelen, S., . . . Lim, K. O. (2007). Neurocognitive and neuroimaging correlates of pediatric traumatic brain injury: A diffusion tensor imaging (DTI) study. *Archives of Clinical Neuropsychology, 22*, 555–568.

Zhang, W., & Buckmaster, P. S. (2009). Dysfunction of the dentate basket cell circuit in a rat model of temporal lobe epilepsy. *Journal of Neuroscience, 29*, 7846–7856.

14

A Summing Up

*In these increasingly competitive times, when the focus of
scientists increasingly turns to research grants, publications,
and academic promotion, let's remember that we all have
come to neurophysiology out of a common desire to
illuminate some interesting problems in the natural
world. Our ultimate goal is not the published paper or the
grant or the promotion, but rather to develop scientific
understanding, a process that is inherently interactive and
self-correcting. . . . Pointing out the caveats, limitations, and
alternative interpretations of your findings is intellectually
honest and a service to the scientific community, not a sign
of weakness. . . . It's rough out there and a little kindness
goes a long way. Remember, we're all striving to reveal
the same truth about neural function—we're all on the
same team.*

—David J. Linden (2008, p.1)

Reviewing Our Intentions

At the outset of this book, we outlined our working hypothesis
that a subtype of PPCS (or mild TBI with persistent symptoms)
can be identified reliably by the presence of multiple intermittent

neurobehavioral symptoms. For lack of an agreed-upon diagnostic label, we chose to call this proposed subtype of PPCS "Multi-symptomatic Intermittent Neurobehavioral Disorder" (or MIND, for short). We reviewed the historical evolution of the description of this neuropsychiatric syndrome by previous experts in the neurobehavioral fields stretching from the seminal writings of psychiatrist Emil Krapelin (Blumer, 2000) to the contemporary work of neurologist Marco Mula (Mula et al., 2010). We also reviewed the existing clinical evidence supporting the use of anticonvulsant mood stabilizers (often in conjunction with SSRI antidepressants) to treat the symptoms of MIND; and we have tried to do so with a realistic sense of the current limitations of that treatment data. We have asserted that MIND is most likely an acquired disorder, with blunt-force head trauma likely to be its most frequent cause in civilian life. We speculated that *some*, but not all, blast-exposed combat veterans with persisting symptoms also may be found to suffer from multiple episodic symptoms. We suggested that MIND patients typically fall in between the cracks between health-care disciplines precisely because they are neuropsychiatric patients with a complex presentation, one that often leads to delayed diagnosis or misdiagnosis. We discussed the manifestations and treatment of this condition in adult patients and in children and adolescents following blunt-force head trauma. We presented behavioral strategies for coping with residual symptoms of MIND when optimal pharmacological treatment leaves an adult patient with residual cognitive and behavioral deficits that continue to be problematic for participating as fully as possible in everyday life. Finally, we tried to address frequently asked questions and unresolved issues regarding MIND as a potentially treatable subtype of PPCS.

Opposition to New Concepts and Paradigms

Having said all that, it is possible that many neuropsychologists and head-trauma experts will question the concept of MIND as a relevant clinical construct for their daily practices. We have observed that progress in clinical science is seldom linear and can be stifled inadvertently by academic orthodoxy or personal biases. For example, it took more than a decade for physicians to accept the proposition that human ulcers were caused by a specific form of bacteria—a breakthrough so important that its proponents ultimately were awarded the Nobel Prize for Medicine in 2005 (Heath & Heath, 2008).

Nonscientists are encouraged to believe that the acceptance of new research and the development of new clinical paradigms are unaffected largely by scientific biases and professional politics within the healthcare community. This view of science is somewhat idealized, however, given that some influential leaders and experts in a field may have vested interests in maintaining the *status quo*.

In the words of educational theorists Heath and Heath (2008): "The best way to get people's attention is to break their existing schemas" (p. 79). We have tried in writing this book to express our views in a manner that is both *credible* and *influential*. However, we anticipate that the proposition that MIND represents an identifiable and treatable subtype of PPCS will run counter to the cognitive schemas of many practicing clinicians, particularly those in the subdiscipline of forensic neuropsychology (i.e., those practitioners who spend a good deal of time testifying in adversarial court procedures and, thus, have inordinate needs to appear right and orthodox on every professional issue).

Probable Skeptics Regarding MIND

Currently, the prevailing belief regarding PPCS among practicing neuropsychologists in the United States is that underlying neurological or brain-related factors seldom play more than a minor role in initiating the clinical presentation of mild TBI patients known as the "miserable minority" (e.g., Grieffenstein, 2009; Heilbronner et al. 2009; Howe, 2009; McCrea et al., 2009; Tsanadis et al., 2008). In that sense, the present book clearly presents a minority report on some unexpectedly poor, clinical outcomes for individuals with persistent, mild TBI or PPCS. We clearly believe that there is a subset of PPCS patients for whom underlying neurological factors may be *primary* and whose symptoms potentially are treatable with mood-stabilizing medications that have anticonvulsant properties. However, our observations and reasoning clearly pose a challenge to the cognitive schemas of experts who hold contrary points of view.

We also believe in the concept of full disclosure and, therefore, intentionally have provided the list of references in the previous paragraph precisely to make it easier for readers to sample other points of view. Accordingly, we encourage care providers, patients, their families, and especially students in training (who hopefully are not yet burdened by rigid belief systems) to read widely in the area of mild TBI and PPCS and to *draw their own conclusions.*

Whether the evidence we have cited in support of our views will be replicated, extended, refuted, ultimately accepted, or substantially transformed by other investigators, only time will tell. In the meantime, it is *not* our intention to encourage widespread iatrogenic disease. It is, however, our intention to redirect clinical attention to a little-known, but often described, neuropsychiatric syndrome, one that may be of direct relevance to assessing and treating some *but not all* patients in the "miserable minority" following blunt-force TBI.

Closing

We believe that postulating the existence of MIND as a treatable subtype of PPCS can help to generate a number of testable hypotheses with regard to improving the assessment and treatment of individuals with mild TBI. As we approach the final chapters of our clinical careers, we eagerly await the accretion of relevant data from other clinicians and other laboratories. We encourage care providers and researchers to consider the material in the following technical appendices.

We close with a quotation from C. Miller Fisher, one of the pre-eminent neurologists of the 20th century. This passage comes from a summary of Fisher's clinical aphorisms by neurologist Louis Caplan (1982):

> Fully accept what you have heard or read only when you have verified it yourself. Whenever possible, test the ideas of others before embracing them as valid or quoting them. The literature and dogma of medicine are filled with hearsay, half-truths, and imaginings. Misinformation and poorly tested "facts" are frequently passed along in rote fashion from one generation to the next. (p. 389)

References

Blumer, D. (2000). Dysphoric disorders and paroxysmal affects: Recognition and treatment of epilepsy-related psychiatric disorders. *Harvard Review of Psychiatry, 8,* 8–17.

Caplan, L. (1982). Fisher's rules. *Archives of Neurology, 39,* 389–390.

Godin, S. (2010). *Linchpin: Are you indispensable?* Boston, MA: Little Brown.

Grieffenstein, M. F. (2009). Clinical myths of forensic neuropsychology. *Clinical Neuropsychologist, 23,* 286–296.

Heath, C., & Heath, D. (2007). *Made to stick: Why some ideas die and others survive.* New York, NY: Random House.

Heilbronner, R. L., Sweet, J. J., Morgan, J. E., Larrabee, G. J., Millis, S. R., Conference Participants. (2009). American Academy of Clinical Neuropsychology Consensus Conference Statement on the neuropsychological assessment of effort, response bias, and malingering. *Clinical Neuropsychologist, 23,* 1093–1129.

Howe, L. L. (2009). Giving context to post-deployment postconcussive-like symptoms: blast-related potential mild traumatic brain injury and comorbidities. *Clinical Neuropsychologist, 23,* 1315–1337.

Linden, D. J. (2008). Warm, fuzzy feeling. *Journal of Neurophysiology, 100*, 1.

McCrea, M., Iverson, G. L., McAllister, T. W., Hammeke, T. A., Powell, M. R., Barr, W. B., & Kelly, J. P. (2009). An integrated review of recovery after mild traumatic brain injury (MTBI): Implications for clinical management. *Clinical Neuropsychologist, 23*, 1368–1390.

Mula, M., Jauch, R., Cavanna, A., Gaus, V., Kretz, R., Collimedaglia, L., . . . Schmitz, B. (2010). Interictal dysphoric disorder and periictal dysphoric symptoms in patients with epilepsy. *Epilepsia*, E-pub ahead of publication.

Tsanadis, J., Montoya, E., Hanks, R. A., Millis S. R., Fichtenberg, N. L., & Axelrod, B. N. (2008). Brain injury severity, litigation status, and self-report of postconcussive symptoms. *Clinical Neuropsychologist, 24*, 1080–1092.

APPENDIX

I

The Iowa Interview

If you do not ask the right questions, you do not get the right answers. A question asked in the right way often points to its own answer. Asking questions is the A-B-C of diagnosis. Only the inquiring mind solves problems.

—Edward Hodnett
(http://thinkexist.com/quotes/edward
_hodnett/ Downloaded 09/12/2010)

Background

This appendix represents a technical resource for health-care providers who potentially are interested in evaluating their patients or clients for symptoms of MIND and for researchers interested in testing hypotheses raised in this book. The Iowa Interview has gone through several iterations, and the development of the interview is discussed at length in Roberts et al. (1990). The current version of the Iowa Interview and normative observations on healthy young adults without histories of brain injury (n = 115) have been published in Roberts (1999).

Head trauma patients and their family members are discouraged actively from self-administering this interview for several reasons. Use of the Iowa Interview by untrained laymen is likely to lead to erroneous conclusions based on incorrect interpretations of item-content. Such an attempt to self-diagnose may lead to false expectations and disappointment on the part of the patient or family. In addition, presenting the "results" of self-diagnosis to one's care provider may produce skepticism or interfere with the development of the longer term doctor-patient relationship. In general, patients with histories of head trauma and their families should be able to determine whether the concept of MIND has potential relevance to their life situations after reading the first five or six chapters of this book. Although information on several earlier versions of the Iowa Interview already has been in the public domain for a number of years, attempted self–administration of the Iowa Interview also may provoke criticism from care providers who are particularly worried about the inadvertent creation of iatrogenic conditions. This may be of special concern if there is pending or possible litigation over the effects of an instance of head trauma.

In the material in this appendix, individual items are discussed in the order in which they are listed on the actual interview form in a previous chapter by R. J. Roberts (1999) on "Epilepsy Spectrum Disorder." (For all intents and purposes, the concept of MIND presented in this book is highly similar to that of Epilepsy Spectrum Disorder presented in Roberts's (1999) previous chapter. However, the acronym MIND was chosen in part to avoid the implication that this proposed subtype of PPCS was necessarily a form of epilepsy.) Items 1 through 17 are grouped together as intermittent psycho-sensory symptoms. Items 18 through 32 constitute intermittent cognitive symptoms. Items 33 through 36 are regarded as episodic affective (i.e., emotional) symptoms. Finally, the last four items, 37 through 40, constitute a small group of residual items having to do with sleep phenomena and daytime sleepiness.

The word "illusion" frequently is used to describe psycho-sensory items. Technically speaking, an illusion is the distortion of a sensory stimulus that actually exists and is perceived, but in an altered fashion; whereas, a hallucination is the false perception of a physical stimulus when none actually exists in the physical environment. Semantic purists will note that many of the "illusions" in the content of the interview are perhaps better regarded as unformed or simple hallucinations. However, we have chosen to use the word "illusion" to minimize possible linkage between symptoms of MIND and symptoms of the primary psychoses, such as schizophrenia and mania, in which hallucinatory experiences are generally much more complex and much more disturbing.

For convenience, a comprehensive listing of the symptom items to be discussed is presented in Table I–1.

Intermittent Psycho-Sensory Symptoms

1. Olfactory Illusions

These are a fairly common symptom for MIND patients. They are generally brief, most often lasting a few seconds to 10 minutes or so. The illusory smells reported by MIND patients are almost always subjectively foul or unpleasant, and the interviewer should be somewhat skeptical of elaborately described positive aromas (e.g., the fragrance of an exotic perfume, the smell of a newly mown lawn "like the green, green grass of home"). Nevertheless, occasional patients with conventional temporal lobe epilepsy report olfactory illusions that are pleasant or neutral (Acharya, Acharya, & Luders, 1998). Although illusory odors of fecal matter, urine, body odor, and "something burning" are commonly reported negative odors, sometimes MIND patients will explain that the odor they smell is "foul" or "nasty" but "indescribable." This type of response should not necessarily be regarded as evasive because brief olfactory illusions or hallucinations do not always have a compelling one-to-one correspondence with specific odors in real life.

The interviewer should make sure that there is no obvious cause for the olfactory illusion in the patient's environment at the time it occurred (e.g., a cat litter box) and should confirm that

Table I-1. Individual Symptom Items from the Iowa Interview (IIPSS)

Type of Symptom	Content of Individual Items
Psycho-sensory	Olfactory Illusions
	Gustatory Illusions
	Illusions of Movement
	Visual Illusions
	Illusions of Shadowy Creatures
	Haptic (Tactile) Illusions
	Episodic Numbness/Tingling
	Episodic Tinnitus
	Auditory Illusions
	Sick Headaches
	Episodic Cephalic Pain
	Illusion of Urinary Urgency
	Micropsia
	Macropsia
	Episodic Dizziness
	Episodic Vertigo
	Epigastric Sensation
Cognitive	Speech Problems
	Word-Finding Lapses
	Speaking Jargon
	Confusional Spells
	Environmental Distortion
	Jamais Vu
	Déjà vu
	Memory Gaps
	Discontinuous TV Viewing
	Automatic Driving
	Unrecalled Behaviors
	Visual Fixation
	Staring Spells
	Mental Decline
	Loss of Consciousness

Table I-1. *continued*

Type of Symptom	Content of Individual Items
Affective	Dysphoric Spells
	Panic/Anxiety Spells
	Temper Outbursts
	Unrecalled Anger
Nocturnal/Sleep Phenomena	Parasomnias
	Irresistible Sleepiness
	Nocturnal Sweating
	Nightmares with Nocturnal Sweating

From: Roberts, R. J. (1999). Epilepsy Spectrum Disorder in the context of mild traumatic brain injury. In N. R. Varney & R. J. Roberts (Eds.), *The evaluation and treatment of mild traumatic brain injury* (pp. 409–447). Mahwah, NJ: Lawrence Erlbaum.

other people in the immediate area do not smell the odor. Occasionally, a patient with olfactory hallucinations (when asked about their sense of smell in a general, open-ended fashion) will reply, "It's too good," suggesting an acute sense of smell; however, upon further inquiry, such a patient often will go on to explain that their sense of smell is so "good" because they can "smell things that other people cannot smell."

If the examiner actually has tested the patient's sense of smell and found such a patient to be totally anosmic, it is still possible for such patients to report experiencing olfactory illusions. It is also important to differentiate olfactory illusions from olfactory flashbacks in traumatized individuals. With olfactory flashbacks, an actual odor in real-life suddenly triggers the re-experiencing of some traumatic memory. For example, a Vietnam veteran with severe PTSD crossed over the U.S./Mexican border and, when he smelled the ambient odors from an impoverished village, he began to replay aversive memories from Vietnam in his mind, became hyper-vigilant, and told his spouse he wanted to leave the village at once. This is a classic example of a patient with PTSD having an olfactory flashback, in that the patient's wife also smelled the unpleasant odors redolent in the impoverished village. It is logically possible to have both olfactory illusions and olfactory-triggered flashbacks, but the presence of both phenomena in a single patient is relatively rare in our clinical experience. More detailed information on olfactory hallucinations and auras in traditional forms of epilepsy can be found in Daly (1975) and Acharya and colleagues (1998).

2. Gustatory Illusions

Like olfactory illusions, illusions of taste are almost always of a bad or foul taste. Illusions of taste usually are described as bitter, sour, or metallic—and quite often as "indescribable." More demonstrative patients will simply say, "it tastes like crap." When pressed, they usually say that the taste they experience is like what they would imagine crap would taste like.

Interviewers should make sure that there is no apparent reason for the presence of a bad taste (e.g., smoking, gastric reflux, waking up with "morning breath," etc.). Often patients will report brushing their teeth or drinking water in an effort to send the illusion away, but these strategies are not successful. Simply having a dry sensation in one's mouth without a true bad taste does not qualify to be scored, as many medications (e.g., tricyclic antidepressants, allergy medications) can produce such dry mouth or "cotton-mouth." Most often in MIND patients, olfactory and gustatory illusions occur separately rather than occurring simultaneously. Information on gustatory hallucinations in the context of traditional epilepsy is presented by Hausser-Hauw & Bancaud (1987).

3. Illusions of Movement (in Vision)

Quite frequently, patients with MIND report seeing the illusion of a shadowy-type figure off the side of their peripheral vision, but, when they turn their heads to the side to check the illusion out, they generally conclude that there was "really nothing there." This visual illusion or unformed hallucination is variously described as being "just movement," "like a shadow," or "a figure, like a person." It also has been described in the traditional epilepsy literature as a "sensed presence" (Persinger & Tiller, 2008). Some patients cope by actively suppressing their attention to such unformed hallucinations after they have experienced it on multiple occurrences

This illusion can be distressing particularly to traumatized combat veterans who are already hyper-vigilant to potential threats to their safety as part of PTSD. Some patients with both PTSD and MIND actually may start to check for an intruder the first few times they experience this symptom. The illusion may occur exclusively just to one side of vision, or it may occur separately off to both sides of peripheral vision. When this happens, the illusion usually occurs with greater frequency off to one side or the other. When the illusion occurs just off to one side, it may be regarded as a "soft" lateralizing sign suggestive of dysfunction in the contralateral hemisphere. Asking about this item sometimes may elicit content about item 5; when it is the case that the patient complains of a small animal-like figure off to one side, score that as positive for item 4 only, rather than being positive for both this item and item 4.

Item 3 also may be described occasionally as the feeling of a "sensed presence," of a different person off to one side of vision or the other. This sensed presence may be interpreted by some patients are having religious or spiritual significance; however, in our experience, more MIND patients tend to experience this illusion of a sensed presence as unpleasant and anxiety-provoking (particularly those with co-morbid PTSD). Some MIND patients have shared that this symptom has made them feel like they were "going psychotic," or words to that effect. If this should occur, it is a good time to offer bland reassurance that many individuals experience brief illusions and to point out the distinction between *being crazy* and *feeling like you are being driven crazy* by symptoms that are out of one's control. Additional information regarding the illusion of a sensed presence in the context of brain injury and epilepsy is available in the clinical literature (Landt-blom, 2006; Persinger, 1994; Persinger & Tiller, 2008; Zijlmans et al., 2009).

4. Visual Illusions

A number of MIND patients experience brief displays of indistinct shape of stars, bugs, snake-like objects, or threads moving in their field of vision, especially in peripheral vision. [These need to be distinguished from "floaters" in the vitreous portion of the eye, on the one hand, and black and white images of beads or bullets that move and are associated with orthostatic hypertension (i.e., blood draining from the brain when one stands up or changes posture too quickly).] Such illusory light shows may last a few seconds or several minutes. They may occur more in one field of vision than the other. More information on visual auras and unformed visual illusions in the context of traditional epilepsy can be found in Taylor, Scheffer, and Berkovic (2003) and Elliott, Joyce, and Shorvon (2009).

5. Illusions of Shadowy Creatures (in Vision)

In addition to the visual illusions described for items 3 and 4, MIND patients also may report experiencing seeing a small creature like a mouse, rat, or small cockroach appearing to scurry across the floor or up a wall (e.g., Liebman & Rodriguez, 2009). When asking about this item, it is important to satisfy oneself that a given patient's residence (e.g., rural farmhouse, poorly kept urban apartment) does not normally have such infestations, that the patient is indeed experiencing a false perception. If the interviewer is seriously in doubt and the responses to follow-up questions do not resolve this doubt, the conservative thing to do with any symptom on the interview is to score it as a "0" (never, or not in the past year) and simply move on to the next item.

It is important to remember that patients may complain of episodic visual disturbance or auras in the context of migraine (e.g., Sjaastad, Bakketeig, & Petersen, 2006). If a clear correlation is described between intermittent visual symptoms and either the prodromal or active phase of migraine pain, consideration should be given to neurologic referral if the patient complains of severe headaches and has not already been evaluated for migraine headaches.

6. Haptic (Tactile) Illusions

This symptom is reported with somewhat lower frequency by MIND patients compared with most of the other intermittent, psychosensory symptoms. Paresthesias are described "as if bugs were crawling" over a body part for brief period of time, or as if something were brushing up against a part of the body, such as a cobweb; however, these false sensations occur for *no apparent reason*. Most of the time, these sensations will be described as occurring on the limbs. Before this item can be scored definitively, the interviewer needs to make sure that the paresthesias are not due to some other cause (e.g., peripheral neuropathy due to diabetes or alcohol abuse, peripheral injury to the nerves of a limb, effects of poor peripheral circulation, previous back injury, etc.). Thus, this item is somewhat more easily interpreted in younger patients who lack the cumulative effects of multiple, chronic, systemic diseases. If the interviewer cannot rule out other causes, or if the sensations reported are described as chronic and static (rather than intermittent or episodic), then the conservative course of action is to score this item as "0" (never, or not in the past year).

7. Episodic Numbness

The same caveats applied to item 6 also apply to item 7. The interviewer should make sure that any numbness reported is intermittent and cannot be attributed to other causes (e.g., such as sitting on top of one's own leg with the circulation cut-off).

Sometimes patients will describe legitimate episodes when the numbness is mixed with a tingling sensation or "like pins and needles." The interviewer should stress the words "*for no apparent reason*" regarding the loss of sensation when reading this item. Information on somatosensory symptoms (such as those covered by items 6 and 7) in the context of traditional epilepsy has been summarized by Erickson, Clapp, Ford, & Jabbari (2006) and Tuxhorn (2005).

8. Episodic Tinnitus

Tinnitus (i.e., ringing in the ears) is an auditory phantom sensation experienced when no such external sound is actually present. Tinnitus may be either episodic (intermittent) or constant. For administering and scoring this item, we are interested in obtaining frequency ratings on *episodic* tinnitus.

The reason for this is because *constant* tinnitus is often peripheral in origin (i.e., reflecting dysfunction at the level of the ear) and, by definition, occurs every day. Constant tinnitus of peripheral origin often is associated with hearing loss due to a variety of causes (e.g., excessive noise exposure, blast injury, exposure to toxic organic solvents, effects of aging, etc.). (Although it may be possible for highly experienced specialists to determine that a given patient has both constant and episodic components to his overall tinnitus profile, making such a determination with accuracy exceeds the judgment of most interviewers.) If a patient or their medical records indicates that the tinnitus is "constant," it is best to score this item conservatively as a "0" (never, or not in the last year) while making a notation as to why this was done. Such a conservative approach also should be taken if the patient suffers from Meniere's disease, a disorder of the inner ear.

Another form of *episodic* tinnitus, however, that is of central origin in the brain, sometimes is called "retrocochlear" (beyond the level of the cochlea) by audiologists. Episodic tinnitus of central origin may occur in only one ear (Hurst & Lee, 1986), or it may be bilateral (Devinsky, 2003). Both ears may ring simultaneously or at separate times. When *episodic* tinnitus occurs only from one auditory channel, it can be a fairly good lateralizing sign for dysfunction in the contralateral hemisphere. Patients with MIND may describe their subjective experiences as intermittent "ringing," "buzzing," "like white noise," "like a high-pitched tone" from an audiometer, or even "a chirping noise." At first some patients may say that it is too difficult to estimate the frequency of such spells because they have tried to disregard them; however, with some reflection and encouragement, such patients usually can provide an estimate of the frequency of these auditory spells.

In our clinical experience, some audiologists may not comment on the central versus peripheral distinctions in clinical reports, even though anticonvulsant agents can be prescribed frequently for tinnitus patients (Smith & Darlington, 2005). Tinnitus is among the most frequent auditory complaints in patients with traumatic brain injury (Lew, Jerger, Guillory, & Henry, 2007), and it may reflect either the effects of diffuse axonal injury to central auditory pathways or the effects of electrical instability in the brain (Fincham, Yamda, Schottelius, Hayreh, & Damasio, 1979). Attias and colleagues discuss the complexities central tinnitus following TBI in greater detail (Attias, Zwecker-Lazar, Nageris, Keren, & Groswasser, 2005). Emerging research findings also have begun to suggest that the brain may exert more of a central modulating effect on many types of tinnitus (Kraus, Ding, Zhou, & Salvi, 2009).

9. Auditory Illusions of the Telephone Ringing

This auditory illusion is reported rather infrequently. Yet, the decision was made to keep the item in the interview because, when it is reported, it is almost always a valid sign of MIND in that it tends to be accompanied by other episodic symptoms. This item also should be scored if the patient mentioned that they thought the doorbell was ringing, but, when they get up to check, no one was there. Occasionally, the patient spontaneously may report that the have heard someone "calling their name." This type of self-report is scored as a "0" for the purposes of the interview, but may be investigated informally by follow-up questions to rule out frank psychosis.

10. Sick Headaches

The classification and treatment of headache following traumatic brain injury (and blast exposure) have been the subject of many articles in and of itself (e.g., Packard, 2000; Hurley, 2009). For the purposes of the Iowa Interview, we emphasize that the headache at least must be associated with nausea or a "sick feeling;" however, actual vomiting is *not* required to score this item positively. Obvious chronic, muscle-tension headaches that pre-existed the acute head trauma, that are brought on only by aversive environmental stimulation (e.g., noisy children shouting), or that are mild enough to obtain good response to use of over-the-counter remedies generally are *not* considered "sick" headaches unless they progress to the point of nausea, for the purposes of the interview. Often a patient will report that he or she has more than one type of headache. In that case, interviewers should have the patient base his answer only on "sick" headaches rather than other types. Physician-verified migraine or vascular headaches, which either started or were markedly intensified following head trauma or blast exposure, should contribute to the overall frequency estimate. If the patient begins to tell the interviewer about *brief* episodes of *abrupt* cephalic pain (see next item), the interviewer should refocus the patient on the extended duration of pain, which constitutes a headache. The patient can be reassured that they shortly will have the chance to describe such brief, discrete episodes of sudden cephalic pain.

Informative reviews of post-traumatic headache have been provided by Hines (1999) and Formisano and his associates (Formisano, Bivona, Catani, D'Ippolito, & Buzzi, 2009) among others. A discussion of headache in the context of traditional epilepsy can be found in Syvertsen, Held, Stovner, and Brodtkorb

(2007). Preliminary studies regarding the onset of persistent headache following blast exposure also have begun to appear in the clinical literature (Hurley, 2009; Neely, Midgette, & Scher, 2009; Ruff, Ruff, & Wang, 2008; Theeler & Erickson, 2009).

11. Episodic Cephalic Pain

In addition to headache problems, MIND patients also report experiencing abrupt episodes of sudden cephalic pain or unusual salient cephalic sensations. Unfortunately, the two of the most common descriptions of such bursts of head pain sound too unusual for some care providers to find them credible. A patient may say, "It feels like a knife or a pin is sticking in the center of my head," or that, "It feels like a jolt of electricity shooting through my head." Despite the florid language, these sensations are usually legitimate symptoms of MIND and *not* reflections of the dramatic presentations of somatizing behavior. Usually, such episodes of cephalic pain are similar to one another from episode to episode. A minority of MIND patients describe painful sensations as moving or shooting from one area of the head to another, either from the occiput forward or from side-to-side.

Such episodes of abrupt cephalic pain typically last from just a few seconds to a couple of minutes at most before the phenomenon subsides. They can be severe enough to temporarily disrupt ongoing behavior ("it brings me to my knees") or to interrupt a patient's train of thought ("What was I saying?"). Facial grimacing may coincide with the onset of such pain. It is not uncommon for the same patient to report clinically significant problems with "sick headaches" (item 10), as well as these much briefer episodes of cephalic pain. Sometimes these briefer episodes may eventually progress to a full-blown "sick" headache (i.e., they may be prodromal to a more extended headache). In this case, it seems reasonable to score both the present item and the preceding item on "sick headaches" on their own merits. More information regarding pain and unusual cephalic sensations in the context of traditional epilepsy can be found in the following sources: Di Bonaventura, Giallonardo, Fattouch, & Manfredi (2004); Manchanda, Freeland, Schaefer, McLachlan, & Blume (2000); Taylor & Lochery (1987); and Van Paesschen, King, Duncan, & Connelly (2001).

12. Illusion of Urinary Urgency

It is a little-known fact that patients with traditional seizure disorders may complain of the false sensation of urinary urgency as a paroxysmal phenomenon (Loddenkemper, Foldvary, Raja, Neme, & Luders, 2003; Baumgartner et al., 2000). Occasionally, patients with MIND also will describe spells of urinary urgency where they try to urinate and "nothing comes out," or there is just a brief dribble that does not seem congruent with the intensity of the felt urge to urinate. If the patient says that this occurs, the interviewer needs to rule out medication-related, prostate-related, and urinary tract-related causes for dysfunction. (Obviously, this item is also easier to interpret in younger, healthy adults.) If there is doubt on the part of the interviewer as to the cause of the reported bouts of illusory urinary urgency, the conservative stance of scoring the item as a "0" (never, or not in the past year) should again be adopted. This item can be endorsed by both men and women.

13. Micropsia

The visual illusion of micropsia occurs when actual objects in the environment are perceived as being smaller than they really are (Taylor, Scheffer, & Berkovic, 2003). Patients also may say that objects appear "farther away" from them than they really are, or they may describe the false perception that the environment appears to be receding or "moving into the distance." This is an infrequently endorsed symptom for patients with MIND. Based upon our clinical experiences, episodic micropsia and its opposite illusion (macropsia) rarely, if ever, co-exist in the same patient.

If the same patient were to endorse both symptoms with clinically significant frequencies, follow-up questions should be employed to convince the interviewer that the patient actually understood the nature of the symptoms they appeared to be endorsing.

14. Macropsia

The visual illusion of macropsia occurs when actual objects in the environment are perceived as being larger than they really are or much closer to the person than they really are. Once again, this is an infrequently endorsed intermittent symptom for patients with MIND. More information on visual illusions associated with a variety of neuropsychiatric syndromes is provided by Norton & Corbett (2000).

15. Episodic Dizziness

Intermittent dizziness reflects subjective instability of the patient without the perception that "the environment is spinning around him." (When the world or room is perceived as spinning around the patient, the symptom is more properly called *vertigo*.) Rarely, there appears to be a visual component with this item involving perceived changes in the surface on which the patient is walking (e.g., "rippling" or "shimmering" of a tiled floor). Episodic dizziness can result from a wide variety of causes. This item refers to episodes of dizziness that occur *"for no apparent reason."* Other conditions (such as circulatory problems, orthostatic hypotension upon standing, Meniere's disease, peripheral vestibular dysfunction, vascular syncope, side effects of medications, and intoxication due to excessive alcohol consumption) are all "apparent reasons" for becoming dizzy, and their effects should not be scored for this item.

Obviously, this individual item is more easily interpreted in younger, healthy adults who have no other causes for bouts of dizziness in their medical histories. On the one hand, there are multiple causes for intermittent dizziness; this would argue against its inclusion on the interview. On the other hand, apparently unexplained and intermittent spells of dizziness occur fairly frequently in MIND patients, and dizziness in general can have important disruptive effects on a patient's life. Dizziness also has been documented to be among the most frequent post-concussive symptoms in the acute phase following head trauma (Yang, Hua, Tu, & Huang, 2009). So the decision was made to retain this symptom on the interview. A more general discussion of dizziness following TBI is provided by Maskell, Chiarelli, & Isles (2006). A summary of the co-occurrence of TBI and vestibular pathology associated with blast exposure has been provided by Scherer & Schubert (2009).

16. Vertigo

Vertigo, for the purposes of this interview, refers to the sensation of having one's environment spinning or whirling around one. Many patients do not actually draw a distinction between dizziness and vertigo in real life (i.e., they tend to lump them both together as "feeling dizzy"), so the interviewer may need to draw this distinction for them. [Most cases of more-or-less chronic vertigo can be divided into benign positional vertigo, labyrinthitis, Meniere's disease, and other types of vestibular disorders (Charles, Fahridin, & Britt, 2008).] For item 16, we are interested only in intermittent bouts of vertigo, which come and go for no apparent reason.

Vertigo, as the sole symptom of a traditionally diagnosed seizure disorder, is thought to be rather rare. Although MIND patients do not report experiencing intermittent vertigo as often as they do intermittent dizziness, it is nevertheless clearly described by some MIND patients as distinct from dizziness. As was also true for episodic dizziness (Item 15), episodes of vertigo due to intoxication do not count when scoring this item. If, after questioning, the interviewer doubts that a given patient has both intermittent dizziness and intermittent vertigo "for no apparent reason," then item 16 should be scored conservatively as "0" (never, or not in the past year). In our experience, it is possible for a MIND patient to legitimately experience both symptoms (i.e., report episodes of both "dizziness" and "vertigo" with clinically significant frequencies).

17. Epigastric Sensation

This intermittent symptom refers to the perceived sensation that one's stomach or internal organs literally are rising up into one's chest or throat. An illustrative analogy can be made to how one feels when a fast elevator ascends very rapidly for a number of floors and then abruptly stops short. Another illustrative analogy can be made to internal sensations felt during a roller-coaster ride. Sometimes MIND patients will describe their epigastric sensations as being associated with flushing or "warmth" in the pit of their stomachs, which then rises up into their chests (e.g., "like a warm ball starting in my stomach and rising up"). Although there also are other types of epigastric sensations and abdominal pains described in the context of traditional forms of epilepsy (Manford & Shorvon, 1992), for the purposes of this interview, we are relying solely upon the description provided here.

Intermittent Cognitive Symptoms

18. Speech Problems

Episodic speech problems refer to intermittent errors in producing coherent speech (even though the person "knows" what it is they want to say linguistically or propositionally). When an interviewer asks about this item, some patients automatically jump to the next two items regarding intermittent problems with language (or linguistic processing) covered by items 19 and 20. If this happens, the patient needs to be redirected back to item 18 and reassured that other language problems will be covered shortly. However, it also is permissible to go with the patient to cover items 19 and 20 on language functioning and then return to item 18. [The important issue is not adhering rigidly to the order of the interview questions, but maintaining the rapport and empathy necessary to obtain accurate information.]

Common intermittent, speech problems described by patients with MIND include episodes of garbled speech, episodes of slurred speech, and the abrupt onset of stammering or stuttering (in an individual with no history of a developmental speech disorder). Unlike many intermittent symptoms of MIND, episodic speech problems can be observed directly by other people, and some patients may have been told by others (or even teased) when they exhibit spells of poor articulation. A number of otherwise normal individuals are markedly phobic about public speaking, and disruption of speech due to anxiety over formal, public speaking (Iverach et al., 2009) should *not* be scored if this is the only time when speech problems emerge.

Generally speaking, MIND patients with intermittent speech articulation problems usually experience such problems in more than one setting (e.g., work versus home; school versus play) and when speaking to more than a single individual (unless there is *extreme* social isolation). There is almost always conscious recognition on the part of the symptomatic person that errors in articulation have occurred. Transiently dysarthric speech has been documented in the context of traditionally defined epilepsy (Gabr, Luders, Dinner, Morris, & Wylie, 1989; Isnard, Guenot, Sindou, & Maugiere, 2004).

19. Word-finding Lapses

As opposed to the problems of motor speech production described in item 18, word-finding lapses refer to the failure of many MIND patients to retrieve the word they want to say from their internal lexicon. Therefore, word-finding lapses generally reflect an intermittent *linguistic* failure (as opposed to a transient failure of motor speech production, as described for item 18). However, such word-finding lapses generally occur less frequently in MIND patients than in chronically aphasic patients with more-or-less constant anomia due to gross, structural lesions (Fridriksson, Baker, & Moser, 2009) or in elderly patients with semantic dementia due to atrophy of the anterior temporal lobes (Jefferies & Lambon Ralph, 2006).

Such intermittent word-finding lapses are annoying and embarrassing to some MIND patients, particularly those who work in settings that place great demand on the precision of spoken language (e.g., business settings with multiple face-to-face meetings). MIND patients tend to say that they frequently "draw a blank," know the word they wish to say but can't "get it out," or report that they lost "the thread of their conversation," or have gotten "derailed" in their "train of thought." If such lapses occur with sufficient frequency, MIND patients with the most severe, intermittent, word-finding lapses actually may look to family members or significant others to prompt them, to fill in anomic gaps for them, or to re-orient them to the their own conversations.

However, MIND patients who endorse clinically significantly frequencies of word-finding lapses may still pass conventional, *untimed* measures of confrontation naming such as the Boston Naming Test or Visual Naming from the Multi-Lingual Aphasia Exam. Performing adequately or barely scraping by on naming tests, while complaining about frequent word-finding lapses, does not necessarily mean that a given patient is being untruthful or malingering. This state of affairs exists because performance on structured naming tests is largely dependent upon the state of the brain when naming behavior is sampled. If one samples naming behavior when the brain function of a MIND patient is experiencing transitory interference or sufficient "neural noise" (Hutt, 1972), the patient may well demonstrate word-finding lapses in response to being asked to name line drawings of objects, as well as being anomic during spontaneous conversation. However, when there is no active cerebral interference when naming is formally tested, a MIND patient may well perform within in normal limits.

Such moment-to-moment variability in cognitive performance may be disconcerting for clinical neuropsychologists who believe that, for a neurobehavioral deficit to be "real" (as opposed to exaggerated or feigned), such a deficit should be present each and every time that a given patient's behavior is sampled (e.g., chronic right hemiplegia following a large, left hemisphere stroke in the motor area). However, as we have argued at length elsewhere in this book, variability in behavior, oscillation of cognitive functions, and unexplained emotional lability are inherent hallmarks of the clinical presentation of MIND patients (cf., Taylor, 1999).

The brain areas underlying word-finding difficulties in conventionally diagnosed temporal lobe epileptics have been studied (Trebuchon-Da Fonseca et al., 2009). Case studies have demonstrated that the extent of such anomic lapses in selected patients can be rather specific (Ashcraft, 1993; Ghika-Schmid & Nater, 2003). Conventionally diagnosed temporal lobe epileptics also have been shown to suffer from inter-ictal problems with word-retrieval in between seizure episodes (Mayeux, Brandt, Rosen, & Benson, 1980). Anomia following TBI has been studied by Kerr (1995).

20. Speaking Jargon

This item refers to episodes of disrupted linguistic output in which the patient chooses the wrong word(s) to express his thoughts and uses words other than those he intended to say. Unlike chronic "jargon aphasia" due to structural lesions, in between spells the speech and linguistic expression of MIND patients with this symptom can appear to be unremarkable. However, during a spell, they may substitute a single inappropriate word (e.g., "bring me a cup of *corn* to drink"). They may use neologisms, make paraphasic errors, or speak "jargon" during an entire sentence or two. Patients may be unaware and puzzled that other people appear not to comprehend what is being said, or they may sense that what they are saying is "wrong" somehow and try to correct or gloss-over what they have said, or they simply may stop speaking. During such spells, aural comprehension of other people's speech and conversation generally remains more or less intact.

These spells of speaking jargon typically last a few seconds and generally not longer than a minute. Thus, they are subtle. Following such a spell, expressive language appears to be normal once again. MIND patients with intermittent expressive language problems may or may not have difficulty with repetition tasks such as Sentence Repetition or Digit Span, or short-term verbal memory tasks, depending upon when their ability to repeat language is sampled by the examiner. If the interviewer or examiner notices a passing problem with expressive language in ongoing conversation with the patient, it is quite appropriate to ask a patient whether such a lapse is typical of reported transient problems with expressive language. Certain patients who report experiencing this symptom multiple times on a daily basis may begin to withdraw socially because of worries that they will be thought to be foolish or stupid by others.

Ictal deficits in expressive language function have been described in the context of traditional epilepsy by Bell and colleagues (Bell, Horner, Logue, & Radtke; 1990) and Inoue and his associates (Inoue, Mihara, Fukao, Kudo Watanabe, & Yagi, 1999).

[At this point in discussing language symptoms, we want to share that we recognize that omission of an item having to do with spells of defective auditory comprehension of other peoples' spoken language from the Iowa Interview was an important oversight. Combat veterans with persistent symptoms following blast exposure seem to report a high frequency of "mishearing" or "miscomprehending" conversations with other individuals. In this regard, it is important to note that previous work using electrical stimulation of the auditory cortex has demonstrated "hearing suppression" in human patients (Fenoy, Severson, Volkov, Brugge, & Howard, 2006). Case studies of paroxysmal fluent aphasia have been reported in the epilepsy literature (Knight & Cooper, 1986; Smith Doody, Hrachovy, & Feher, 1992). Thus, although we have no systematic data to present, it seems likely that some

MIND patients experience intermittent spells of receptive language dysfunction much like they experience spells of expressive language dysfunction and episodic word-finding lapses.]

21. Confusional Spells

Fairly commonly, MIND patients will endorse having experienced relatively brief spells of mental confusion without apparent clouding of the sensorium. Such spells may last from 10 to 20 seconds up to 5 or 10 minutes. Confusional spells are described variously as "not being able to get my thoughts together," "blanking out about what I wanted to do next," or going to a different room in the house and "not knowing why I went in there." The onset and offset of bouts of confusion are typically relatively sudden. For patients who are handy with tools, they may get "stuck" in the middle of completing a common task that has multiple steps and unable to figure out what they should do next. One housewife described opening the refrigerator door with a specific purpose seemingly in mind only to stand blankly at the contents of the open refrigerator, unable to recall what it was she intended to do next. During such spells, MIND patients are *not* completely unresponsive, but may act somewhat irritable or "blank" when they are questioned by others. Frequent spells of transient confusion may interfere seriously with vocational or academic performances, particularly when learning new material or demonstrating newly learned material is required. Such spells also can be problematic for individuals doing manual piecework with multiple steps involved (e.g., light assembly factory work or soldering).

Patients with traditional forms of epilepsy may experience confusion prior to a seizure, during a partial seizure, or postictally following a seizure (Gnanamuthu, 1988). When mental confusion due to unrecognized, nonconvulsive *partial status epilepticus* (a term for an extended seizure that does not spontaneously resolve) is prolonged, the cognitive effects can be so severe that the dysfunction can be mistaken for dementia in the elderly

(Tombini et al., 2005). In children, confusion and incomplete awakening in the middle of the night occasionally may be due to a frank seizure disorder (Davey, 2009). During the daytime, children with epilepsy may be identified incorrectly as manifesting symptoms of ADHD by their teachers or parents (Dunn & Kronenberger, 2005).

22. Environmental Distortion

This item describes episodes when the surrounding environment (or the "world" around a person) suddenly appears weird, strange, or distorted somehow, as if the patient had "entered the twilight zone" for a brief period of time. For example, one middle-aged golfer with a history of head trauma described how one day the third hole at his home course "just didn't look right, not the way it should." When he played the same whole the next day, it once again looked like it always had. Such spells usually are associated with felt anxiety, emotional uneasiness, or intellectual puzzlement. Episodes when such spells are associated with the use of illicit drugs should be ignored for the purposes of the interview and not scored. For administering and scoring this item, the change in perception is emphasized (as opposed to the intense inner conviction associated with *jamais vu*, as will be described in the following section). If an interviewer believes that there is substantial overlap between this item and *jamais vu* as described in item 23, then only one of the two items should be included in the total score generated by the interview, in order to err on the side of being conservative.

Various types of metamorphopsia (visual distortions of a perceived object or scene in the environment) in the context of traditional forms of epilepsy have been described by Elliott et al. (2009).

23. *Jamais Vu*

This phrase from the French literally means "never seen" before and applies to situations in which places or people that should look familiar to the patient appear as if they are being seen for the first time. Episodes of *jamais vu* typically are accompanied by a sense of fear or eeriness. Subjective, internal conflict often exists between what the patient "perceives" and the inner conviction regarding what that patient cognitively "knows to be true." *Jamais vu* has long been known to be a symptom of temporal epilepsy (or partial seizure disorders) and initially was identified as an epileptic symptom by Hughlings Jackson, one of the giants of 19th century neurology. Jackson classified it as one of the "dreamy states" due to epileptic activity (Sengoku, Toichi, & Murai, 2005). In both traditional epileptics and MIND patients, *jamais vu* is a symptom that is reported considerably less frequently than the opposite symptom *déjà vu*. In the context of MIND, patients will report that for a period of time the appearance of normally familiar person or a well-known street scene simply "doesn't look the way it should." Occasionally, a patient may feel the need to pull off the road and scrutinize landmarks, trying to make sure he or she is, in fact, driving on their intended route—even though it is a route they may have taken numerous times.

A crucial distinction between an episode of *jamais vu* and a dissociative flashback (due to psychological trauma) is that the patient does *not* feel removed from the present time and place with *jamais vu*, as tends to be the case with severe flashbacks. With *jamais vu*, the patient remains in the present; with a severe, dissociative flashback, the patient reports feeling that their sense of time has separated subjectively from the present or that they have been "transported" both in time and geographic location (e.g., "It felt like I was back in Vietnam all over again.").

24. Déjà vu

Vernon Neppe, a neuropsychiatrist, has described *déjà vu* as a subjectively inappropriate impression of familiarity of a present experience with an experience that did not actually occur in the past (Neppe, 1983). One might describe *déjà vu* as an "experiential" illusion. *Déjà vu* is a common enough experience in neurologically normal human beings that most healthy people have experienced it one or more times. However, *déjà vu* in the context of cerebral dysfunction often is accompanied by extremely unpleasant feelings of dread or anxiety during the episode (Wild, 2005). Because many neurologically normal individuals report experiencing nonpathological *déjà vu*, this item tends not to be very discriminating as a single symptom on the Iowa Interview.

Gloor [1991, cited in Wild, 2005,] has written extensively on the anatomy of *déjà vu* and other experiential phenomena in temporal lobe epilepsy, as have Bancaud and colleagues (Bancaud, Brunet-Bourgin, Chauvel, & Halgren, 1994). Sadler and Rahey (2004) recommend that care be taken to separate *déjà vu* from what they described as the "aura of prescience." Prescience refers to the subjective feeling or "precognition," the subjective conviction that one knows what is going to occur in one's environment in the immediate future. In contrast, *déjà vu* refers to the illusory feeling that one already has experienced an event or a situation at some time in the past. Both prescience and *déjà vu* can occur in the context of traditional temporal lobe epilepsy; however, prescience refers to feelings regarding the future, whereas *déjà vu* relates to a fictitious past event that seems to be re-occurring in the present. For the purposes of the Iowa Interview, instances of prescience should not be regarded by the interviewer as contributing to the score on item 24.

25. Memory Gaps

Many MIND patients will endorse experiencing brief memory gaps during which they cannot remember anything that happened around them for a period of time up to five minutes or so. In most instances, such patients appear to others to be in touch which their environment (and may even be directly responsive to other people), but later on, it is recognized that the memory structures in the brains of the MIND patients were not encoding information deeply enough that it could be stored efficiently for later retrieval (Glowinski, 1973). Accordingly, this item represents the first of four items (25 through 28) that are directed at assessing brief periods of transient *recent memory failure*. Devoting four separate items to various types of memory lapses and memory gaps was deemed appropriate because complaints of "poor memory" following mild TBI are one of two symptoms that are most bothersome to the patients themselves (the other being frequent, severe headaches). Memory lapses have been an underexplored topic in neuropsychological research in general, and even highly detailed reviews of memory dysfunction (e.g., Budson, 2009; Meador, 2007) often completely neglect the topic of discrete memory lapses. [This oversight is unfortunate because the technology needed to investigate the neural bases of brief mental lapses has been evolving rapidly (Weissman, Roberts, Visscher, & Woldorff, 2006). Similarly, the capacity of patients to retrieve information when they need it and to recall future intentions in a timely fashion, so-called "prospective memory," also has been a relatively neglected topic until just the past few years (e.g., Tay, Ang, Lau, Meyyappan, & Collinson, 2009).]

For item 25, it is important to emphasize to the patient that "day-dreaming" (i.e., intense inward focus with active mentation) should not count toward the frequency estimate to be provided by the patient. This is because, when one is daydreaming, one can later recall the content of one's daydream and explain it to another person in great detail. Also, falling asleep or napping for a few minutes does not count toward the frequency estimate for this item. Similarly, the intense preoccupation associated with cognitive or visual intrusions associated with severe PTSD should not contribute to the frequency estimate on this item. As is true for daydreams, cognitive intrusions or "day-mares" (which are associated with reduced processing of environmental stimulation in the present) should not count toward scoring this item. Neither should other clearly dissociative phenomenon such as a prolonged "flashback," "losing time" for one or two days, or experiencing an extended fugue state. If an interviewer is unsure how to regard a certain patient's answer to this item, it is appropriate to ask follow-up questions, such as: "How do you know that you have these brief memory gaps?" or "Are you actively concentrating on other thoughts during this period of time," or "Is your mind best described as being 'blank'?"

As is true for word-finding lapses (item 19), some clinicians act as if they believe all memory problems must be (a) demonstrable on formal testing; and (b) replicable from one assessment to the next, or from one test to the next within an assessment, in order for a memory defect to be considered "real" or "genuine." However, some individual MIND patients who endorse having frequent memory lapses can perform reasonably well on formal tests of short-term learning of new information, whereas other MIND patients will score below expectations on such memory tasks based upon their obtained level of general IQ. Furthermore, within the 3 to 4 hours minimally required for most neuropsychological exams, patients may perform adequately for much of the exam, but then develop a brief confusional spell or experience an extended memory lapse later on in the exam, or *vice versa*. This is a major reason why both authors try to administer or observe major portions of a neurobehavioral exam, as opposed to relying solely upon testing technicians. Such cognitive lapses can be "real" but fairly subtle, if one does not have sufficient clinical experience with such transitory neurobehavioral phenomena to recognize them when they occur.

Once again, it needs to be emphasized that *the outcomes on neuropsychological testing or mental status screening depend upon the state of the patient's brain function at the time the assessment of memory is conducted* (e.g., Benton, 1984; Manes, Hodges, Graham, & Zeman, 2001). Stated another way, if brain function is relatively normal when a given behavior or cognitive function is sampled by the examiner, then performance should be relatively normal; on the other hand, if the patient's brain is less than fully functional when a behavior or cognitive function is sampled, then there is likely to be test-based evidence of transitory cognitive impairment. [For neurologically normal individuals, the performance of everyday tasks can vary tremendously at different times within the same person depending on the specific circumstances (Hedden & Gabarieli, 2006). We would argue that variability of complex cognitive performances on tests is likely to much more variable, however, for patients with MIND-like symptoms than for healthy control subjects (e.g., Mintz, et al., 2009).]

Clinical research from epileptologists has demonstrated that discrete periods of memory dysfunction can be associated with episodes of electrophysiological dysfunction in patients with traditional forms of epilepsy (Butler et al., 2009). In their words,

> Transient epileptic amnesia (TEA) is a recently recognised form of epilepsy of which the principle manifestation is recurrent, transient episodes of isolated memory loss. In addition to the amnesic episodes, many patients describe significant inter-ictal memory difficulties. (p. 357)

Even relatively brief, subclinical, seizure activity can disrupt the demonstration of new learning on commonly used neuropsychological tasks, such as list-learning (Bridgman, Malamud, Sperling, Saykin, & O'Connor, 1989) and reaction time (Aldenkamp, Beitler, Arends, vander Linden, & Diepman, 2005; Shewmon & Erwin,1988).

Some clinicians regard "transient epileptic amnesia" (TEA) as a distinct clinical syndrome (Butler et al., 2007; Gallassi, 2006), one that is probably under-recognized and under-diagnosed (Mendes, 2002). Other neurologists, however, have expressed skepticism regarding the existence of TEA and suggested that over-use of the concept could lead to excessive prescription of anticonvulsant medications in middle-aged and elderly patients (Stirano, Zara, & Striano, 2007; Bilo, Meo, Ruosi, de Leva, & Striano, 2009). What does seem clear, however, is that brief memory lapses clearly do occur in *some* conventionally epileptic patients (Weiss & Spiegel, 2008; Manes, Hodges, Graham, & Zeman, 2001).

Some researchers have speculated that brief memory lapses (in the context of otherwise adequate cognition and behavior) might be due to the effects of "subclinical" discharges in the brain (Gallasi, 2006). For example, Kasteleijn-Nolst Trenite & Vermeiren (2005) have demonstrated previously that "subclinical epileptiform discharges" (SEDs) as short as 0.5 seconds can interrupt ongoing cognitive processing. (It has become a standard practice in parts of Europe to screen air traffic controllers with EEG methods for the presence of brief cognitive lapses associated with abnormal electrical discharges in the brain.)

Although there are ample precedents from the traditional epilepsy research literature for patients having discrete memory lapses and memory gaps, much of this work has been conducted in Europe. The phrase "transitory cognitive impairment" (TCI) has been used by European epileptologists since the mid-1980s to describe the disruption of ongoing cognitive performances in epileptic patients by subclinical, inter-ictal EEG changes (i.e., discharges that could be identified on standard EEG but did not result in overt observable seizures). Because much of the work on TEA and TCI has been performed in Europe and published in journals devoted primarily with epilepsy, this body of work may be relatively less familiar to North American clinicians who deal predominantly with TBI. (To support this speculation, a Medline computer search on the intersection of "traumatic brain injury and transitory cognitive impairment" produced no useful references on intermittent symptoms following brain injury.) Nevertheless, patients with MIND frequently report feeling socially handicapped or vocationally impaired by transitory memory gaps and sudden cognitive lapses.

26. Discontinuous TV Viewing

This item also is directed at eliciting self-report of memory gaps. When administering this item, make sure to emphasize that daydreaming and falling asleep on the couch in front of the TV do not count as true "gaps" in memory. Patients who always watch TV alone may report losing the thread of the plot in a movie or having to replay the video cassette or DVD in order to fill in gaps in the plot. Sports fans may report that they may have missed a discrete portion of a timed sporting event. For example, a football fan may recall the two-minute warning before halftime, and the next thing he subsequently recalls is both teams heading into the locker rooms at the end of the half. Patients with frequent, brief memory gaps who watch TV with other viewers may bother others with repeated questions about what's going on in the plot of a movie or TV show because the patient has "spaced off" and lost the thread of the action. In the extreme instances, a patient with MIND may even have given up watching TV because it is too frustrating to tolerate frequent or extended memory lapses while doing so.

27. Automatic Driving

This is a rather infrequently endorsed item for MIND patients, but one that is qualitatively quite striking when it is reported. In administering the item, it is sometimes difficult to make the content of the item distinct from extended, subjective preoccupation (i.e., inward-focus) that often accompanies driving: normally occurring "highway hypnosis" (Cerezuela, Tejero, Choliz, Chisvert, & Manteagudo, 2004). Many normal drivers experience stretches of long-distance driving on an uncrowded super-highway when they appear to go into a light trance with an internal focus of attention (e.g., trying to solve some problem or formulating some future plan). However, they continue to operate the motor vehicle fairly automatically and routinely arrive at their appointed destination. If normal individuals are interrupted in such an inner-focused state, they can tell a fellow passenger what they had been thinking about. However, MIND patients with automatic driving report a more extreme, frustrating, and sometimes worrisome state of affairs. They tend to sail past exits and turn-offs, even on familiar routes; they may end up at destinations they had not intended upon (e.g., supermarket rather than the local lumberyard), or they suddenly may become aware that they have been heading in an entirely different direction than from the one they planned to travel. Interestingly enough, virtually all MIND patients we have interviewed have reported that they apparently continued to operate their motor vehicles safely during such episodes. Conscientious car drivers and professional vehicle operators (e.g., long-haul truck drivers), however, tend to become worried appropriately about the future implications of this symptom, after they realize that they have apparently engaged in an extended episode of unrecalled "automatic driving." Children and adolescents with MIND-like symptoms (who are not old enough to drive) blankly may wander the halls at school between classes or bicycle to places they normally would not go in an unfocused manner for no apparent reason.

28. Unrecalled Behaviors

This item requires that the patient report on feedback from other people regarding things that the patient has supposedly said or done—but that he or she has later failed to recall. [If we were to do things over again with full foresight, we might possibly have limited this item solely to unrecalled conversations because (1) such unrecalled conversations appear to be the most frequent exemplars of this item; and (2) such unrecalled conversations tend to create relationship issues of varying severity for patients with MIND and their significant others.] Occasionally, a patient will start some task only to find that they previously had started it (or even finished it) and could not recall having even worked on it previously. More frequently, a patient will fail to remember part or all of a conversation in which they seemed to be participating sensibly at the time, but when they apparently did not encode the experience with sufficient depth to permit later retrieval. Spouses, family members, co-workers, and close friends frequently contend that the patient did indeed engage in such conversations, and arguments can become frequent enough and sufficiently vehement to rupture social relationships. One spouse may accuse the other spouse of repeatedly blowing them off; bosses may accuse workers of having failed to follow explicit instructions on the job site. In fact, simply asking a patient this question in the presence of a significant other occasionally precipitates a major disagreement during an office interview. Efforts should be made to tone down such adversarial conversations before they become outright arguments in the clinician's office.

In a study of symptoms that can occur following TBI, Gordon and colleagues found that *unrecalled behavior* was one of the symptoms that was most sensitive to and specific for TBI patients when a wide range of neurobehavioral symptom occurrence was studied in various groups of clinical patients (Gordon, Haddad, Brown, Hibbard, & Silwinski, 2000). In their work with traditional epilepsy patients, Butler & Zeman (2008) have emphasized that recurrent memory lapses " . . . can have a profound impact on patients' lives," in part because "their presence goes undetected by standard memory tests . . . " (p. 2243).

29. Visual Fixation

This is the first of two consecutive items designed to assess the possible presence of brief staring spells. (This item asks patients to report on their own subjective experiences, whereas item 30 asks patients to report on what other people have told them about the presence of staring spells.) Some MIND patients tend to become unintentionally fixated on bright or shiny objects (or some random stimulus, like a spot on the wall) and keep their unbroken gaze directed to that point to the exclusion of other ongoing stimuli. This sort of episode usually is described as a passive, almost trance-like, but involuntary experience (spellbound). It may not be particularly distressing while it is occurring, and patients typically report little or no voluntary desire to break their gaze away. Fixating like this typically is accompanied by subjective "blankness" rather than by daydreaming, active mentation, extreme preoccupation, or anxiety.

While the patient is visually fixated, motor behavior generally is inhibited (Fromm, 1986), and such spells are *not* accompanied by the obvious motor automatisms of traditional complex partial seizures (e.g., lip-smacking, eye-blinking, picking at one's clothes). A visually fixated patient may be slow to respond verbally if they are addressed by someone else during this period of time. Intentional eyes-open visual fixation associated with voluntary meditation practice does *not* count for patients who practice such mindfulness techniques for purposes of relaxation or self-control.

30. Staring Spells

Even though TBI patients may report being unaware of staring spells, other people in their social environments may still observe brief periods of time when MIND patients are staring off and do not appear to be fully in contact with the surrounding environment. Some observers may actually inquire whether a patient is "okay" at such times. If the patient himself denies ever having been told about staring spells, but the significant other reports observing obvious staring spells, then the interviewer should ask the significant other how frequently such staring spells tend to occur, and this item should be scored according to the report of the significant other. Sometimes brief staring spells have been witnessed so frequently by the friends or family of a MIND patient that they may have adopted a nickname for the patient (e.g., "space cadet," "air-head") or a pet phrase for the spells themselves (e.g., "Tower to Earth, tower to Earth, come in Earth?"). During such spells, the content of the patient's mind usually is described as having been "blank."

If a significant other asks what a MIND patient was thinking about during an apparent lapse, a patient typically may say, "Nothing," or make up some seemingly plausible answer to deflect further inquiry. In classroom situations, children mistakenly may be thought to be manifesting the "inattentive subtype" of Attention Deficit Disorder by their teachers. For adults with combat-related PTSD, staring spells may seem qualitatively similar to the "1000-yard stare" of the traumatized combat veteran; however, when such a staring episode is associated with cognitive intrusions or extreme preoccupation, PTSD patients retain the capacity to tell someone else about the events that were being recollected (although they may consciously elect to keep the matter private and not wish to share it anyone); in contrast, MIND patients generally report *the absence of active cognition* during a staring spell.

Distinguishing features of epileptic and nonepileptic staring spells in children are discussed at length by Rosenow and colleagues (Rosenow et al., 1998).

31. Mental Decline (Scored Dichotomously)

This is the only item from the Iowa Interview that is scored on a dichotomous "0" versus "6" basis. If the patient responds that they feel like their memory and concentration are getting worse as time goes by, the item is scored as a "6." If they report that memory and concentration are staying the same or even improving as time passes (e.g., as a result of being prescribed an SSRI medication for depression), then the item is scored as a "0." It has been our experience that untreated, adult MIND patients subjectively regard their subjective memory and concentration functioning as getting worse with the passage of time, although we lack systematic data to support this clinical observation empirically. However, some cognitive functions (e.g., dichotic listening performance) may improve, or even normalize, in association with positive symptomatic response to treatment with anticonvulsant mood-stabilizers (Roberts, 1999).

32. Loss of Consciousness

This item is seldom endorsed by MIND patients, unless they have another medical condition that produces unconsciousness (e.g., vasovagal fainting, drop attacks); however, item 32 was retained on the Iowa Interview because of its general importance for the diagnosis and management of the health of individual patients. Loss of consciousness is striking as a symptom and occurs for a variety of reasons, many of them serious. Yet, it is surprising that many individuals who have experienced loss of consciousness do not seek prompt medical evaluation (Setnik & Bazarian, 2007). If the patient knows why they lost consciousness (e.g., syncope), then the item is scored as a "0," if the cause of the spell appears unrelated to the effects of head trauma. Loss of consciousness due to excessive ingestion of drugs or alcohol also should be excluded from consideration. Although not technically part of the interview, it is always appropriate to ask whether the patient sustained additional head trauma or other injuries when they lost consciousness. (Loss of consciousness due to hypoxia associated with myocardial infarction might itself be a cause of MIND-like symptoms in patients without histories of head trauma.)

If a patient reports multiple unexplained instances of loss of consciousness following head trauma, it is possible that they may have developed some type of conventional seizure disorder (Blumenfeld, 2005; Cavanna & Monaco, 2009; Pedley, 1983; Thijs, Bloem, & van Dijk, 2009; Yu & Blumenfeld, 2009). If it has not already been accomplished, prompt neurologic consultation should be sought.

Intermittent Affective Symptoms

33. Dysphoric (Depressive) Spells

It is clear from the clinical literature on traditional epilepsy that both seizure discharges in the brain and artificial electrical stimulation of the brain can produce abrupt changes in mood or "mood swings" (Blumer, 2000; Elliott, Joyce, & Shorvon, 2009a; Gloor, Olivier, Quesney, Andermann, & Horowitz, 1982). Just as an unformed hallucination is a *percept without a stimulus*, a spell-like change in mood can be experienced *in the absence of an obvious eliciting stimulus in the environment* (Blumer, 2000; Williams, 1956). In the words of Williams:

> . . . by popular usage an hallucination, which is a percept without a stimulus, may be organic or psychotic. An

organic hallucination occurs when through brain disease [or dysfunction] the patient has a percept without a stimulus, into the nature of which he usually has insight. Local disturbance of the brain has evoked a perceptual response. . . . But percepts may arise within the body—be proprioceptive as well as exteroceptive, and there can be no fundamental difference between sensations felt in a limb or through the eye as a result of a local epileptic discharge . . . for the physiological changes in the cerebrum responsible for both are highly similar. They can all be considered organic hallucinations, caused by the epileptic discharge. . . . The feelings [that is "mood-states"] called fear, depression or pleasure arising in the attack [also] have no local reference; in other regards they are similar, and for physiological purposes can be considered to be hallucinations. (p. 32)

Even the first systematic study of epileptic auras recognized that at least 5% of auras were "psychical" in nature (Gowers, 1901).

Unfortunately, there is no commonly accepted term to describe such a "rogue" mood-state, one that automatically intrudes upon human consciousness as if it had a "will of its own." The phrase "ictal depression" implies that such a mood-state could be associated only with a conventional type of epileptic seizure. The phrases "ego-alien" or "ego-dystonic" depression both carry with them unwanted psychodynamic implications. Describing such spells as "square-wave" bouts of depressed mood may be useful for scientifically inclined patients (e.g., engineers), and it permits the interviewer to draw an illustrative diagram, but doing so may just be confusing with less scientific patients. Perhaps the most poetic and apt description of the concept of a depressive spell was provided to us by a highly verbal patient of ours who complained of " . . . episodes of depressed mood that came *unbidden*." Blumer (2000), a prominent epileptologist, has employed the phrase "paroxysmal affect" to describe this type of emotional spell as an inter-ictal complication of traditional forms of epilepsy. However, Blumer (2000) also noted that such "paroxysmal affects" can occur in apparently nonepileptic individuals with other medical conditions (e.g., migraine).

Most of us believe that when we experience an intense emotional experience or sudden affective state that we must be doing so "for some reason," that we should be aware of a conscious link between the intensely felt affect and the nature of the external stimuli or internal thoughts associated with our strong change in emotional tone. It can be threatening for some patients (and a few care providers), to consider the possibility that a malfunctioning human brain can produce abnormal emotions in consciousness as a by-product of neuronal misfiring. Almost all human beings strive to "make sense" of the events in their lives. However, in order to make sense of unexplained, intense, paroxysmal affects, some patients will construct erroneous misattributions (e.g., "I must have had too much coffee today," or "That's my PTSD kicking up again") as plausible explanations for puzzling spells of strong emotion. This tendency of our brains to attempt to fill in apparent meaning where there is none has been called "confabulation" in its most extreme forms. Because this is a characteristic human tendency (often made more pronounced by TBI), it is crucial for clinical interviewers to listen very closely to the phenomenology of patient symptoms (and their subjective complaints, such as those on the Iowa Interview), but to not necessarily accept the patient's reasoning as to *why* a particular symptom is present. Listen to patients' symptoms carefully, but question patients' attributions as to why their symptoms occur.

Many patients with MIND report a chronic low-level depression or "dysthymia" (Blumer, Monouturis, & Davies, 2004; Roberts, 2008), as well as discrete periods of time when their moods become abruptly more unhappy "for no apparent reason." In that case, it is better to describe this change as an abrupt *worsening* of mood because their baseline affect is somewhat dysphoric to begin with. Patients with histories of severe psychological trauma and strong dissociative tendencies also may experience periods of ego-dystonic depression, and such moods may be difficult for even experienced interviewers to distinguish from similar spells in the context of MIND. Rather than sticking slavishly to the exact wording of item 33 on the interview form, the interviewer may need to find additional ways to communicate the abruptness of onset, the absence of a known eliciting event in consciousness, or the equally mysterious offset of a depressive spell after a period of time ranging from 5–10 minutes, to several hours, up to a couple of days.

In the words of Blumer et al. (2005),

> These pleiomorphic dysphoric episodes occur without external triggers and without clouding of consciousness. They begin and end rapidly and recur fairly regularly in a uniform manner, lasting from a few hours up to 2 days. . . . A patient just awakens with the dysphoria, or it develops insidiously through the course of a day. (p. 828)

For a minority of MIND patients, a depressive spell may become so intense that they feel like crying or began to notice suicidal ideation. As with all patients, the clinician needs to take steps to keep the patient safe if there is acute suicidal ideation or an abrupt flare-up of semi-chronic suicidal ideation.

In the words of Bortz (2003), "Depression [as a syndrome] occurs so frequently in patients with epilepsy that screening for major mood disorder is routine in the clinical examination of patients with medically refractory seizures." (p. 781). A case study of a patient with temporal lobe epilepsy who experienced depressive spells has been presented by Ros (2004), who labeled such phenomena "dysthymic attacks" (p. 161). Blumer (2000) also has discussed cases of "subictal dysphoric disorder" in the context of epilepsy. Similarly, a wide range of abrupt affective changes in children with partial seizure disorders has been reported by Fogarasi, Janszky, & Tuxhorn (2007).

34. Panic/Anxiety Spells

Among traditionally diagnosed temporal lobe epileptics, intermittent episodes of untriggered anxiety or fear are even more common than intermittent episodes of depressed mood. Once again, the focus of this item is on a mood-state that comes over the patient suddenly *for no apparent reason*. The literature on conventional epilepsy indicates that intense, ictal fear may be even the main (or sole) feature of a partial seizure disorder (Biraben et al., 2001; Huppertz, Franck, Korinthenberg, & Schulze-Bonhage, 2002).

Furthermore, fear episodes due to limbic seizures may occur with normal, ictal, scalp EEG results (Devinsky, Sato, Theodore, & Porter, 1989). There are some data suggesting that the amygdala of the right (nondominant) hemisphere may be preferentially involved in ictal fear responses (Sazgar, Carlen, & Wennberg, 2003). Other findings suggest that the orbito-frontal and temporal structures both need to be activated in order to produce intense, ictal states of fear or anger (Bartolo-meil et al., 2002). Further complicating matters clinically, it is possible for epileptic patients to experience panic attacks as a primary psychiatric disorder unrelated to their seizures (Mintzer & Lopez, 2002; Spitz, 1991). Also, psychologically trau-matized individuals with severe PTSD and other dissociative disorders may sometimes experience panic episodes that appear to come "out of the blue," as if traumatic affect has been dissoci-ated or split off from full memory recall of an entire traumatic event.

After item 33 has been administered successfully, it usually becomes easier for the person being interviewed to understand the intent of item 34. The essential features are similar for both items: (a) the onset of the spell of anxiety or fear is abrupt; (b) there is no apparent eliciting stimulus or "trigger" in the environment; and (c) the offset of the mood is equally as inexpli-cable as the onset. If patients have been treated successfully for primary Panic Disorder in the past with antidepressant medica-tions, it is best to score this item conservatively as "0" (never, or not in the past year), unless the patient indicates that a qualita-tively different type of anxiety spell has emerged following an intervening instance of TBI.

35. Temper Outbursts

This appears to be the MIND symptom that most distresses the family members of head-trauma patients. In the words of Blumer (2000),

> The interictal outbursts of angry affects that were commonly noted by pre-modern psychiatrists still present a frequent problem among the patients seen today. The outbursts rarely occur in the physician's office, and next-of-kin often will not report the trouble, particularly in the presence of the patient. Their occurrence should be explored as part of the inquiry for other dysphoric symptoms, because the entire disorder is well treatable by pharmacological intervention. The irritable dysphoric episodes tend to show a characteristic pattern. The patients are not completely overwhelmed by their furious excitement during the outbursts and are able to harness their behavior; the attack remains verbal, is directed against inanimate objects, avoids harmful injury to others, and is followed by genuine remorse. After a period of hours, patients will revert to their more customary good-natured selves. . . . Typically, the family is concerned about this troublesome "Jekyll and Hyde" behavior but remains supportive of the patient. Episodes of rage lasting days are uncommon. (pp. 15–16)

From our experiences with MIND patients, we agree with Blumer that, in most instances, the expression of such outbursts is solely verbal. However, some patients may throw objects close at hand (e.g., dishes, tools, etc.), or punch drywall with their fists to the point of bruising their knuckles. Generally, any such destruction of personal property seems random rather than focused clearly upon hurting or intimidating other people. When a MIND patient comes to their senses after the fact, they may be genuinely apologetic or act appalled by the extent of their emotional explosion (Taylor, 1999). Many men with symptoms of MIND often may meet DSM-IV-TR criteria for the diagnosis of Intermittent Explosive Disorder (Coccaro, Posternak, & Zimmerman, 2005) in our experience. If there is physical aggression on the part of a MIND patient, it usually is "impulsive" or "irritable" in nature, as opposed to premeditated or clearly directed toward the self-serving goal of controlling other people (Stanford, Houston, & Baldridge, 2008). Another way of thinking about irritable aggression is that the angry individual seems to have a hair-trigger temper, which is too easily provoked by situational factors; however, the behavioral expression of such irritability later evokes guilt and shame on the part of the patient. In contrast, the successful perpetrator of premeditated, operant aggression usually seems quite pleased or feels rewarded when an intentional violent display (e.g., willfully shooting the family's pet dog to make a point about discipline) successfully exerts control over the immediate social environment (Stanford, Houston, Mathias, Villemarette-Pittman, Helfritz, & Conklin, 2003). (However, because a single patient can manifest more than just one type of anger-disorder, an irritable individual with symptoms of MIND may, at other times, also employ operant aggression or manipulative expressions of anger in order to bully others into getting their way.)

Although the exact wording for item 35 stresses becoming "extremely and intensely angry *for no reason*," MIND patients also are likely to exhibit excessive reactivity to relatively trivial events (e.g., yelling incoherently at full volume for several minutes after a preschool-aged child accidentally spills a glass of milk). In other words, the response is way out of proportion to the provocation. Also, sometimes MIND patients report that they simply "wake up" in a highly irritable mood some mornings for no apparent reason.

Some patients with better insight into their irritability try to isolate in order decrease the potential for social conflict after they sense they are at increased risk of becoming irritable. Some spouses of MIND patients report that the identified patient may get a "certain look" in their eyes immediately prior to a rage outburst, one that serves as a warning to the family to retreat from possible confrontations.

The conventional wisdom from the literature on traditional epilepsy is that true ictal violence is rather rare (Treiman, 1991; Summer, Atik, Unal, Emre, & Atasoy, 2007). Anger displays more often have been thought to be reactions to attempted restraint of an epileptic patient by other people or to be "post-ictal" in nature, reflecting ongoing epileptic confusion and faulty processing of social cues. An interesting and extensive case study involving "multimodal" evaluation of an epileptic patient with aggression has been provided by Poprawski and colleagues (Poprawski et al., 2007).

Recently, epileptologists using intracerebral recording techniques have proposed that ictal emotional disturbances, including facial displays of rage involve underlying, transient "loss of synchrony" between the orbital-frontal cortex and the amygdala (Bartolomei et al., 2005). Essentially, their notion is that seizure activity emanating from the frontal lobes can disrupt normal mechanisms of emotional regulation located in part in subcortical structures within the temporal lobes.

Within the past decade, there has been increased interest in "anger attacks" and Intermittent Explosive Disorder on the part of biological psychiatrists in the context of studying affective disorder. In the words of Posternak and Zimmerman (2002), "Anger and aggression are prominent in psychiatric outpatients to a degree that may rival that of depression and anxiety; it is therefore important that clinicians routinely screen for these symptoms" (p. 665). Similarly, Coccaro and colleagues found that "intermittent explosive disorder is a much more common condition than previously recognized" (Kessler et al., 2006). Although most studies have found a higher rate of anger attacks for men, women also are subject to such anger attacks followed by guilt and remorse (Mammen et al., 1999.) Although relatively little is known about the etiology of anger outbursts, it has been suggested that they may be variants of existing affective disorders (Fava, Anderson, & Rosenbaum, 1990). Others researchers cite evidence implicating both psychological trauma and witnessed violence (Fincham et al., 2009), as well as a history of mild traumatic brain injury (Amara, Richa, & Bayle, 2007; N. Gordon, 1999) as possible contributing factors.

Studies of brain-injured individuals have substantiated that irritable aggression can be a significant clinical problem for both adults and children (Brower & Price, 2001; Dooley, Anderson, Hemphill, & Ohan, 2008; Greve et al., 2001). It also is noteworthy that both carbamazepine and divalproex have been used successfully to treat extreme irritability and outbursts in brain-injured individuals in the absence of conventional seizures (Anderson, 2008; Blumer, Heilbronn, & Himmelhoch, 1988; Lux, 2007).

36. Unrecalled Anger

Rarely, the families of MIND patients report that the patient has had an anger spell in which he did not seem to recollect the spell afterwards, leaving him puzzled as to why family members would still be upset with him. During spells of rage that are later unrecalled, patients sometimes are described as "glassy-eyed," "not making sense," or partially (but not fully) out of contact with their surroundings. Typically, such an unrecalled spell just gradually resolves in a matter of minutes, or occasionally the patient complains of feeling "tired" afterward and may lie down to take a nap. As is true for working with all types of patients, care must be taken to address family safety issues, in addition to diagnosing and treating the identified patient.

Nocturnal/Sleep-Related Phenomena

37. Parasomnias

Parasomnias are disruptive sleep-related disorders (Mahowald, 2004). This general term encompasses sleep-walking and sleep-talking, restless legs (and arms) syndrome, and periodic leg movements. In one of our cases, a patient arose from sleep, urinated in a trashcan in the bedroom rather than using the toilet in the bathroom, and went back to bed. In another case, the patient got up, apparently opened the refrigerator door, went back to bed, and the next morning accused his spouse of having left the door open all night. A normally behaved, eight-year-old boy was found cutting up the family drapes with scissors in the middle of the night with a confused look on his face, and he failed to recall the episode when he awakened the next morning.

Sometimes nocturnal events are so distressing that a spouse may choose to sleep in a different room. Such dramatic but pointless behavior in the midst of a sleep-cycle may represent the effects of a so-called "REM sleep behavior disorder" (Mahowald & Schenck, 2009). In normal rapid eye movement (REM) sleep, the relative generalized paralysis that normally accompanies dreaming is absent, so a patient may appear to be acting out their dreams with yelling, talking, grabbing, flailing their limbs, or even punching (Crompton & Berkovic, 2009). Combat veterans with PTSD may report that they have nonsensically hit, kicked, or even choked a spouse in the middle of a sleep cycle (Husain, Miller, & Carwile, 2001).

Although we currently lack systematic data, it seems likely that MIND patients describe more frequent and strange nocturnal phenomena in the midst of the sleep-cycle than do neurologically normal individuals. It is fairly well-established that individuals with traumatic brain injury are at increased risk for developing sleep disorders across the broad spectrum of severity of TBI (Castriotta et al., 2007).

Certainly not all sleep disorders are associated with the presence of MIND. For instance, when asking about this item, *it is good clinical practice to also use the opportunity to inquire about possible sleep apnea syndromes*. This is because the coexistence of untreated sleep apnea in MIND patients may worsen overall behavioral functioning during the daytime due to prolonged relative hypoxia at night. Although it is unclear whether sleep apnea is associated specifically with symptoms of MIND, it is important to ask about snoring and breath-holding during sleep in order to ascertain whether clinical referral for a sleep study might be worthwhile. It also is helpful to have access to a spouse or other significant collateral informant when one is asking about snoring or breath-holding spells at night. If a patient resides alone and does not have a regular sleeping partner, it can be helpful for the patient to solicit feedback from other people (e.g., traveling companions) who might have had their own sleep disrupted by the patient's loud snoring. If all else fails, the patient can record their own night-time breathing on a tape recorder for later playback; more than one neurologist or ENT physician has been convinced to pursue a full sleep apnea work-up after listening to an audiotape of manifest snoring with breath-holding spells. Self-arousals due to snoring should not be considered evidence of parasomnia-like behavior and should be excluded from the patient's frequency estimation of this item.

In general, if one frequently is working with neuropsychiatric patients, it is helpful to review the indications for polysomnography and related procedures (Chesson et al., 1997; Malow, Fromes, & Aldrich, 1997). A highly accessible introduction to sleep and its disorders has been provided by Dement and Vaughan (1999).

38. Irresistible Sleepiness

Some MIND patients report experiencing irresistible sleepiness during the daytime and then sleep or nap so profoundly that it is extremely difficult to wake them up. Whether this extreme daytime drowsiness is merely a manifestation of poor sleep at night is unclear. However, it has long been known that brain-injured patients are more easily fatigued following their injuries (Lezak, 1978). Some recent investigators have attributed this loss of energy to increased stress following an injury (e.g., Bay & Xie, 2009); whereas others have suggested that the increased effort to perform cognitive tasks that were more automatic prior to injury may contribute to cognitive fatigue. In some cases, both factors may be operative.

When administering this item, daytime episodes of extreme sleepiness due to intentional lack of sleep, disrupted work schedules, and the effects of recreational or prescription drugs should be excluded. Also, the portion of the item requiring difficulty with subsequent arousal after one has fallen asleep in the daytime should be emphasized. Patients with sleep apnea syndromes and narcolepsy also may complain of excessive daytime sleepiness, and prompt neurological referral may be a consideration, especially if patients report falling asleep at the wheel, while using potentially dangerous tools (e.g., a lathe), or dozing off at a job or school setting where they need to perform well (Pagel, 2009).

Masel and colleagues have discussed the correlates of excessive daytime sleepiness in adults with brain injury (Masel, Scheibel, Kimbark, & Kuna, 2001). The comorbidity of conventional epilepsy and sleep disorders of various types has been explored by Herman (2006) and Malow & Vaughn (2002).

39. Nocturnal Sweating

When asking about this item, be sure to emphasize that there is no clear, environmental cause for the episodes of nocturnal sweating (i.e., the bedroom is not too warm, the patient's sleeping partner has not pushed the covers on top of the patient in the middle of the night, etc.). There are multiple causes for night sweats, so this item should not be attributed to MIND if it is clear that the patient likely has a completely different etiology (e.g., cardiovascular pathology, menopause). Interestingly, a recent, computerized literature search produced no useful, recent references on excessive nocturnal sweating in the context of either TBI or conventional epilepsy. However, the opposite complaint, chilling with "goose bumps," occasionally occurs in the context of nocturnal pilomotor seizures (Ahern, Howard, & Rice, 1988).

40. Nightmares with Nocturnal Insomnia

When administering this item, the interviewer should be sure to emphasize that vivid nightmares are *followed* by abrupt awakening and inability to get back to sleep for at least an hour. Since

PTSD was adopted as a formal diagnosis in 1980, it probably is the first or second diagnosis that comes to mind (along with major depressive disorder) when a mental health professional hears a patient complain about recurrent nightmares or weird, repetitive dreams. However, many neurologists have documented that repetitive and severe nightmares also can be associated with seizure disorders (e.g., Boller, Wright, Cavalieri, & Mitsumoto, 1975; Epstein, 1964; Stewart & Bartucci, 1986; Reami, Silva, Albuquerque, & Campos, 1991; Silvestri & Bromfield, 2004).

Thus, both PTSD patients (presumably without overt seizure discharges) and conventionally diagnosed temporal lobe epileptics may have stereotypical, repetitive dreams that are clinically disturbing to the individual patient. To borrow the words of Stewart and Bartucci (1986), the relationships between temporal epilepsy, PTSD, and dreaming remain "complicated and variable" (p. 113) when assessing patients with significant histories of both psychological trauma and head trauma.

Summary

Like all man-made tools, the Iowa Interview is an imperfect instrument and one that is only as good as the judgment of the clinical interviewer who employs it. With full hindsight, we probably would have deleted some of the existing items or included a few additional items in their place. In the course of inquiring about episodic lapses in linguistic functioning, it is fairly common for MIND patients to report that there are brief periods of time when their aural, receptive language functioning appears to short-circuit for a matter of seconds up to a minute or two. As mentioned previously, this is probably the most conspicuous omission from the version of the Iowa Interview. Also, it almost goes without saying that patients with suspected PPCS or mild TBI should be assessed for suicidal potential. Several recent studies have suggested that persistent mild TBI is associated with increased risk of suicidal ideation and behavior.

If you are a care provider approaching this material for the first time, you may already have asked yourself, "What do such diverse items have in common?" or "Why should such diverse symptoms be included in one interview?" Our best answer, however unsatisfying, is that we hope that the Iowa Interview represents a sort of general "fever thermometer" for detecting the effects of subclinical electrophysiological dysfunction in the human brain. Although a given patient's response to any one item may or may not be of clinical utility in and of itself, the total score on the Iowa Interview hopefully will provide a global measure of cerebral electrical instability, a concept akin to an additional axis on the multi-axial system of DSM-IV-TR.

Whereas EEG evaluation is fairly objective, eliciting self-report on items reflecting the perceived level of electrical stability of the brain is necessarily subjective. As already has been discussed, not every patient who produces an elevated score on the Iowa Interview necessarily suffers MIND due to some form of brain trauma. This is where the *clinical judgment* of the evaluating clinician plays a crucial role in helping to produce efficacious outcomes for the individual patient. Ultimately, the practical utility of any assessment device is only as good as the acumen and consistency of interviewer who administers it and the caliber of the clinician who then interprets the interview results in the context of all other relevant history and diagnostic information.

References

Acharya, V., Acharya, J., & Luders, H. (1998). Olfactory epileptic auras. *Neurology, 51*, 56–61.

Ahern, G. L., Howard, G. F., 3rd, & Weiss, K. L. (1988). Posttraumatic pilomotor seizures: A case report. *Epilepsia, 29*, 640–643.

Aldenkamp, A. P., Beitler, J., Arends, J., van der Linden, I., & Diepman, L. (2005). Acute effects of subclinical epileptiform EEG discharges on cognitive activation. *Functional Neurology, 20*, 23–28.

Amara, G., Richa, S., & Bayle, F. J. (2007). Intermittent explosive disorder: Current status. *Encephale*, *33*, 339–345.

Anderson, R. J. (2008). Shell shock: An old injury with new weapons. *Molecular Interventions*, *8*, 204–218.

Ashcraft, M. H. (1993). A personal case history of transient anomia. *Brain & Language*, *44*, 47–57.

Attias, J., Zwecker-Lazar, I., Nageris, B., Keren, O., & Groswasser, Z. (2005). Dysfunction of the auditory system in patients with traumatic brain injuries with tinnitus and hyperacusis. *Journal of Basic Clinical and Psychological Pharmacology*, *16*, 117–126.

Bancaud, J., Brunet-Bourgin, F., Chauvel, P., & Halgren, E. (1994). Anatomical origin of déjà vu and vivid "memories" in human temporal lobe epilepsy. *Brain*, *117*, 71–90.

Bartolomei, F., Trebuchon, A., Gavaret, M., Regis, J., Wendling, & Chauvel, P. (2005). Acute alteration of emotional behavior in epileptic seizures in related to transient desynchrony in emotion-regulation networks. *Clinical Neurophysiology*, *116*, 2473–2479.

Bartolomei, F., Guye, M., Wendling, F., Gavaret, M., Regis, J., & Chauvel, P. (2002). Fear, anger and compulsive behavior during seizure involvement of large scale fronto-temporal neural networks. *Epileptic Disorders*, *4*, 235–241.

Baumgartner, C., Groppel, G., Leutmezer, F., Aull-Watschinger, S., Pataraia, E., Trinka, E., . . . Bauer, G. (2000). Ictal urinary urge indicates seizure onset in the nondominant temporal lobe. *Neurology*, *55*, 432–434.

Bay, E., & Xie, Y. (2009). Psychological and biological correlates of fatigue after mild-to-moderate traumatic brain injury. *Western Journal of Nursing*, *31*, 731–747.

Bell, W. L., Horner, J., Logue, P., & Radtke, R. A. (1990). Neologistic speech automatisms during complex partial seizures. *Neurology*, *40*, 49–52.

Benton, A. L. (1984). Neuropsychological assessment. In H. I. Kaplan & B. J. Sadock (Eds.), *Comprehensive textbook of psychiatry* (3rd ed., Vol. 1, pp. 520–529). Baltimore, MD: Williams & Wilkins.

Bilo, L., Meo, R., Ruosi, P., de Leva, M. F., & Striano, S. (2009). Transient epileptic amnesia: An emerging late-onset epileptic syndrome. *Epilepsia, 50 (suppl. 5)*, 58–61.

Biraben, A., Taussig, D., Thomas, P., Even, C., Vignal, J. P., Scarabin, J. M., & Chauvel, P. (2001). Fear as the main feature of epileptic seizures. *Journal of Neurology, Neurosurgery, and Psychiatry, 70*, 186–191.

Blumenfeld, H. (2005). Consciousness and epilepsy: Why are patients with absence seizures absent? *Progress in Brain Research, 150*, 271–286.

Blumer, D. (2000). Dysphoric disorders and paroxysmal affects: Recognition and treatment of epilepsy-related psychiatric disorders. *Harvard Review of Psychiatry, 8*, 8–17.

Blumer, D., Heilbronn, M., & Himmelhoch, J. (1988). Indications for carbamazepine in mental illness: Atypical psychiatric disorder or temporal lobe syndrome. *Comprehensive Psychiatry, 29*, 108–122.

Blumer, D., Montouris, G., & Davies, K. (2004). The interictal dysphoric disorder: Recognition, pathogenesis, and treatment of the major psychiatric disorder of epilepsy. *Epilepsy and Behavior, 5*, 826–840.

Boller, F., Wright, D. G., Cavalieri, R., & Mitsumoto, H. (1975). Paroxysmal "nightmares." Sequel of a stroke responsive to diphenylhydantoin. *Neurology, 25*, 1026–1028.

Bortz, J. J. (2003). Neuropsychiatric and memory issues in epilepsy. *Mayo Clinic Proceedings, 78*, 781–787.

Bridgman, P. A., Malamut, B. L., Sperling, M. R., Saykin, A. J., & O'Connor, M. J. (1989). Memory during subclinical hippocampal seizures. *Neurology, 39*, 853–856.

Brower, M. C., & Price, B. H. (2001). Neuropsychiatry of frontal lobe dysfunction in violent and criminal behavior: A critical review. *Journal of Neurology, Neurosurgery, and Psychiatry, 71*, 720–726.

Budson, A. E. (2009). Understanding memory dysfunction. *Neurologist, 15*, 71–79.

Butler, C. R., Bhaduri, A., Acosta-Caronero, J., Nestor, P. J., Kapur, N., Graham, K. S., . . . Zeman, A. Z. (2009). Transient epileptic amnesia: Regional brain atrophy and its relationship to memory deficits. *Brain, 132,* 357–368.

Butler, C. R., Graham, K. S., Hodges, J. R., Kapur, N., Wardlaw, J. M., & Zeman, A. Z. (2007). The syndrome of transient epileptic amnesia. *Annals of Neurology, 61,* 587–598.

Butler, C. R., & Zeman, A. Z. (2008). Recent insights into the impairment of memory in epilepsy: Transient epileptic amnesia accelerated long-term forgetting and remote memory impairment. *Brain, 131,* 2243–2263.

Castriotta, R. J., Wilde, M. C., Lai, J. M., Atanasov, S., Masel, B. E., & Kuna, S. T. (2007). Prevalence and consequences of sleep disorders in traumatic brain injury. *Journal of Clinical Sleep Medicine, 15,* 249–356.

Cavanna, A. E., & Monaco, F. (2009). Brain mechanisms of altered conscious states during epileptic seizures. *Nature Reviews: Neurology, 5,* 267–276.

Cerezuela, G. P., Tejeor, P., Choliz, M., Chisvert, M., & Monteagudo, M. J. (2004). Wertheim's hypothesis on "highway hypnosis": Empirical evidence from a study on motorway and conventional road driving. *Accident Analysis and Prevention, 36,* 1045–1054.

Charles, J., Fahridin, S., & Britt, H. (2008). Vertiginous syndrome. *Australian Family Physician, 37,* 299.

Chesson, A. L., Jr., Ferber, R. A., Fry, J. M., Grigg-Damberger, M. Hartse, K. M., Hurwitz, T. D., . . . Sher, A. (1997). The indications for polysomnography and related procedures. *Sleep, 20,* 423–487.

Coccaro, E. F., Posternak, M. A., & Zimmerman, M. Prevalence and features of intermittment explosive disorder in a clinical setting. *Journal of Clinical Psychiatry, 66,* 1221–1227.

Crompton, D. E., & Berkovic, S. F. (2009). The borderland of epilepsy: Clinical and molecular features of phenomena that mimic epileptic seizures. *Lancet Neurology, 8,* 370–381.

Daly, D. D. (1975). Ictal clinical manifestations of complex partial seizures. *Advances in Neurology, 11,* 57–83.

Davey, M. (2009). Kids that go bump in the night. *Australian Family Physician, 38,* 290–294.

Dement, W. C., & Vaughan, C. (1999). *The promise of sleep*. New York, NY: Dell.

Devinsky, O. (2003). A 48-year-old man with temporal lobe epilepsy and psychiatric illness. *Journal of the American Medical Association, 290*, 381–392.

Devinsky, O., Sato, S., Theodore, W. H., & Porter, R. J. (1989). Fear episodes due to limbic seizures with normal ictal scalp EEG: A subdural electrographic study. *Journal of Clinical Psychiatry, 50*, 28–30.

Di Bonaventura, C., Giallonardo, A. T., Fattouch, J., & Manfredi, M. (2005). Symptoms in focal sensory seizures. Clinical and electroencephalographic features. *Seizure, 14*, 1–9.

Dooley, J. J., Anderson, V., Hemphill, S. A., & Ohan, J. (2008). Aggression after pediatric traumatic brain injury: A theoretical approach. *Brain Injury, 22*, 836–846.

Dunn, D. W., & Kronenberger, W. G. (2005). Childhood epilepsy, attention problems, and ADHD: Review and practical considerations. *Seminars in Pediatric Neurology, 12*, 222–228.

Elliott, B., Joyce, E., & Shovron, S., (2009). Delusions, illusions and hallucinations in epilepsy: 1. Elementary phenomena. *Epilepsy Research, 85*, 162–171.

Epstein, A. W. (1964). Recurrent dreams; their relationship to temporal lobe seizures. *Archives of General Psychiatry, 10*, 25–30.

Erickson, J. C., Clapp, L. E., Ford, G., & Jabbari, B. (2006). Somatosensory auras in refractory temporal lobe epilepsy. *Epilepsia, 47*, 202–206.

Fava, M., Anderson, K., & Rosenbaum, J. F. (1990). "Anger attacks:" Possible variants of panic and major depressive disorders. *American Journal of Psychiatry, 147*, 867–870.

Fenoy, A. J., Severson, M. A., Volkov, I. O., Brugge, J. F., & Howard, M. A. (2006). Hearing suppression induced by electrical stimulation of human auditory cortex. *Brain Research, 118*, 75–83.

Fincham, D., Grimsrud, A., Corrigall, J., Williams, D. R., Seedat, S., Stein, D. J., & Myer, L. (2009). Intermittent explosive disorder in South Africa: Prevalence, correlates and the role of traumatic exposures. *Psychopathology, 42*, 92–98.

Fincham, R. W., Yamada, T., Schottelius, D. D., Hayreh, S. M., & Damasio, A., (1979). Electroencephalographic absence status with minimal behavior change. *Archives of Neurology, 36,* 176–178.

Fogarasi, A., Janszky, J., & Tuxhorn, I. (2007). Ictal emotional expression of children with partial epilepsy. *Epilepsia, 48,* 121–123.

Formisano, R., Bivona, U., Catani, S., D'Ippolito, M., & Buzzi, M. G. (2009). Post-traumatic headache: Facts and doubts. *Journal of Headache Pain, 10,* 145–152.

Fridriksson, J., Baker, J. M., & Moser, D. (2009). Cortical mapping of naming errors in aphasia. *Human Brain Mapping, 30,* 2487–2498.

Gabr, M., Luders, H., Dinner, D., Morris, H., & Wyllie, E. (1989). Speech manifestations in lateralization of temporal lobe seizures. *Annals of Neurology, 25,* 82–87.

Gallassi, R. (2008). Transient epileptic amnesia: Old syndrome or new? *Annals of Neurology, 63,* 409.

Ghika-Schmid, F., & Nater, B. (2003). Anomia for people's names, a restricted form of transient epileptic amnesia. *European Journal of Neurology, 10,* 651–654.

Gloor, P., Olivier, A., Quesney, L. F., Andermann, F., & Horowitz, S. (1982). The role of the limbic system in experiental phenomena of temporal lobe epilepsy. *Annals of Neurology, 12,* 129–144.

Glowinski, H. (1973). Cognitive deficits in temporal lobe epilepsy. An investigation of memory functioning. *Journal of Nervous and Mental Disease, 257,* 129–137.

Gnanamuthu, C. (1988). Confusional states and seizures. When are they related? *Postgraduate Medicine, 84,* 149–152.

Gordon, N. (1999). Episodic dyscontrol syndrome. *Developmental Medicine and Child Neurology, 41,* 786–788.

Gordon, W. A., Haddad, L., Brown, M., Hibbard, M. R., & Sliwinski, M. (2000). The sensitivity and specificity of self-reported symptoms individuals with traumatic brain injury. *Brain Injury, 14,* 21–33.

Gowers, W. R. (1901). *Epilepsy and other convulsive diseases.* Philadelphia, PA: Blackiston.

Greve, K. W., Sherwin, E., Stanford, M. S., Mathias, C., Lovem J., & Ramzinski, P. (2001). Personality and neurocognitive correlates of impulsive aggression in long-term survivors of severe traumatic brain injury. *Brain Injury, 15,* 255–262.

Hausser-Hauw, C., & Bancaud, J. (1987). Gustatory hallucinations in epileptic seizure. Electrophysiological, clinical and anatomical correlates. *Brain, 110,* 339–359.

Hedden, T., & Gabrieli, J.D. (2006). The ebb and flow of attention in the human brain. *Nature Neuroscience, 9,* 863–865.

Herman, S. T. (2006). Epilepsy and sleep. *Current Treatment Options in Neurology, 8,* 271–279.

Hines, M. E. (1999) Posttramatic headaches. In N. R. Varney & R. J. Roberts (Eds.), *The evaluation and treatment of mild traumatic brain injury* (pp. 375–410). Mahwah, NJ: Lawrence Erlbaum.

Huppertz, H. J., Franck, P., Koringthenberg, R., & Schulze-Bonhage, A. (2002). Recurrent attacks of fear and visual hallucinations in a child. *Journal of Child Neurology, 17,* 230–233.

Hurley, D. (2009). Unique clinical, imaging findings seen among veterans with mild TBI. *Neurology Today, 9,* 18–20.

Hurst, R. W., & Lee, S. I. (1986). Ictal tinnitus. *Epilepsia, 27,* 769–772.

Husain, A. M., Miller, P. P., & Carwile, S. T. (2001). REM sleep behavior disorder: Potential relationship to post-traumatic stress disorder. *Journal of Clinical Neurophysiology, 18,* 148–157.

Hutt, S. J. (1972). Experimental analysis of brain activity and behavior in children with "minor" seizures. *Epilepsia, 13,* 520–534.

Inoue, Y., Mihara, T., Fukao, K., Kudo, T., Watanabe, Y., & Yagi, K. (1999). Ictal paraphasia induced by language activity. *Epilepsy Research, 35,* 69–79.

Isnard, J., Guenot, M., Sindou, M., & Mauguierie, F. (2004). Clinical manifestations of insular lobe seizures: A stereo-electroencephalographic study. *Epilepsia, 45,* 1079–1090.

Iverach, L., O'Brian, S., Jones, M., Block, S., Lincoln, M., Harrison, E., . . . Onslow, M. (2009). Prevalence of anxiety disorders among adults seeking speech therapy for stuttering. *Journal of Anxiety Disorders, 23,* 928–934.

Jefferies, E., & Lambon Ralph, M. A. (2006). Semantic impairment in stroke aphasia versus semantic dementia: a care-series comparison. *Brain,* 129, 2132–2147.

Kasteleijn-Nolte Trenite, D. G., & Vemeiren, R. (2005). The impact of subclinical epileptiform discharges on complex tasks and cognition: Relevance for aircrew and air traffic controllers. *Epilepsy and Behavior, 6,* 31–34.

Kerr, C. (1995). Dysnomia following traumatic brain injury: An information-processing approach to assessment. *Brain Injury, 9,* 777–786.

Kessler, R. C., Coccaro, E. F., Fava, M., Jaeger, S., Jin, R., & Walters, E. (2006). The prevalence and correlates of DSM-IV intermittent explosive disorder in the National Comorbidity Survey Replication. *Archives of General Psychiatry, 63,* 669–687.

Knight, R. T., & Cooper, J. (1986). Status epilepticus manifesting as reversible Wernicke's aphasia. *Epilepsia, 27,* 301–304.

Kraus, K. S., Ding, D., Zhou, Y., & Salvi, R. J. (2009). Central auditory plasticity after carboplatin-induced unilateral inner ear damage in the chinchilla: Up-regulation of GAP-43 in the ventral cochlear nucleus. *Hearing Research, 255,* 33–43.

Landtblom, A. M. (2006). The "sensed presence:" An epileptic aura with religious overtones. *Epilepsy and Behavior, 9,* 186–188.

Lew, H. L., Jerger, J. F., Guillory, S. B., & Henry, J. A. (2007). Auditory dysfunction in traumatic brain injury. *Journal of Rehabilitation Research and Development, 44,* 921–928.

Lezak, M. D. (1978). Subtle sequelae of brain damage. Perplexity, distractibility, and fatigue. *American Journal of Physical Medicine, 57,* 9–15.

Liebman, R. F., & Rodriguez, A. J. (2009). A patient with epilepsy and new onset of nocturnal symptoms. *Review of Neurologic Diseases, 6,* 40–44.

Loddenkemper, T., Foldvary, N., Raja, S., Neme, S., & Luders, H. O. (2003). Ictal urinary urge: further evidence for lateralization to the nondominant hemisphere. *Epilepsia 44,* 124–126.

Lux, W. E. (2007). A neuropsychiatric perspective on traumatic brain injury. *Journal of Rehabilitation Research and Development, 44,* 951–962.

Mahowald, M. W. (2004). Parasomnias. *Medical Clinics of North America,* 88, 669–678.

Mahowald, M. W., & Schenck, C. H. (2009). The REM sleep behavior disorder odyssey. *Sleep Medicine Review, 13,* 381–384.

Malow, B. A., Fromes, G. A., & Aldrich, M. S. (1997). Usefulness of polysomnography in epilepsy patients. *Neurology, 48,* 1389–1394.

Malow, B. A., & Vaughn, B. V. (2002). Treatment of sleep disorder in epilepsy. *Epilepsy and Behavior, 3*(5S), 35–37.

Mammen, O. K., Shear, M. K., Pilkonis, P. A., Kolko, D. J., Thase, M. E., & Greeno, C. G. (1999). Anger attacks: Correlates and significance of an underrecognized symptom. *Journal of Clinical Psychiatry, 60,* 633–642.

Manchanda, R., Freeland, A., Schaefer, B., McLachlan, R. S., & Blume, W. T. (2000). Auras, seizure focus, and psychiatric disorders. *Neuropsychiatry, Neuropsychology, and Behavioral Neurology, 13,* 13–19.

Manes, F., Hodges, J. R., Graham, K. S., & Zeman, A. (2001). Focal autobiographical amnesia in association with transient epileptic amnesia. *Brain, 124,* 499–509.

Manford, M., & Shorvon, S. D. (1992). Prolonged sensory or visceral symptoms: an under-diagnosed form of non-convulsive focal (simple partial) status epilepticus. *Journal of Neurology, Neurosurgery, and Psychiatry, 55,* 714–716.

Masel, B. E., Scheibel, R. S., Kimbark, T., & Kuna, S. T. (2001). Excessive daytime sleepiness in adults with brain injuries. *Archives of Physical Medicine and Rehabilitation, 82,* 1526–1532.

Maskell, F., Chiarelli, P., & Isles, R. (2006). Dizziness after traumatic brain injury: Overview and measurement in the clinical setting. *Brain Injury,* 20, 293–305.

Mayeux, R., Brandy, J., Rosen, J., & Benson, D. F. (1980). Interictal memory and language impairment in temporal lobe epilepsy. *Neurology,* 30, 120–125.

Meador, K. J. (2007). The basic science of memory as it applies to epilepsy. *Epilepsia, 48 (suppl.),* 23–25.

Mendes, M. H. (2002). Transient epileptic amnesia: An under-diagnosed phenomenon? Three more cases. *Seizure, 11*, 238–242.

Mintz, M., Legoff, D., Scornaienchi, J., Brown, M., Levin-Allen, S., Mintz, P., & Smith, C. (2009). The underrecognized epilepsy spectrum: The effects of levetiracetam on neuropsychological functioning in relation to subclinical spike production. *Journal of Child Neurology, 24*, 807–815.

Mintzer, S., & Lopez, F. (2002). Comorbidity of ictal fear and panic disorder. *Epilepsy and Behavior, 3*, 330–337.

Neely, E. T., Midgette, L. A., & Scher, A. I. (2009). Clinical review and epidemiology of headache disorder in US service members: With emphasis on post-traumatic headache. *Headache, 49*, 1089–1096.

Neppe, V. M. (1983). *The psychology of déjà vu: Have I been there before?* Johannesburg, South Africa: Witwatersrand University Press.

Norton, J. W., & Corbett, J. J. (2000). Visual perceptual abnormalities: Hallucinations and illusions. *Seminars in Neurology, 20*, 111–121.

Packard, R. C. (2000). Treatment of chronic daily headache with divalproex sodium. *Headache, 40*, 736–739.

Pagel, J. F. (2009). Excessive daytime sleepiness. *American Family Physician, 79*, 391–396.

Pedley, T. A. (1983). Differential diagnosis of episodic symptoms. *Epilepsia, 24*(Suppl. 1), S31–S44.

Persinger, M. A. (1994). Sense of a presence and suicidal ideation following traumatic brain injury: Indications of right-hemispheric intrusions from neuropsychological profiles. *Psychological Reports, 75*, 1059–1070.

Persinger, M. A., & Tiller, S. G. (2008). Case report: A prototypical spontaneous "sensed presence" of a sentient being and concomitant electroencephalographic activity in the clinical laboratory. *Neurocase, 14*, 425–430.

Poprawski, T. J., Pluzaczka, A. N., Chennamchetty, V. N., Halaris, A., Crayton, J. W., & Konopka, L. M. (2007). Multimodality imaging in a depressed patient with violent behavior and temporal lobe seizures. *Clinical EEG and Neuroscience, 38*, 175–179.

Posternak, M. A., & Zimmerman, M. (2002). Anger and aggression in psychiatric outpatients. *Journal of Clinical Psychiatry*, 2002, *63*, 665–672.

Reami, D. O., Silva, D. F., Albuquerque, M., & Campos, C. J. (1991). Dreams and epilepsy. *Epilepsia, 32*, 51–53.

Roberts, R. J. (1999). Epilepsy Spectrum Disorder in the context of mild traumatic brain injury. In N. R. Varney & R. J. Roberts (Eds.), *The evaluation and treatment of mild traumatic brain injury* (pp. 409–447). Mahwah, NJ: Lawrence Erlbaum.

Roberts, R. J. (2008, December–January). Impact on the brain. *Scientific American Mind*, 50–57.

Roberts, R. J., Varney, N. R., Hulbert, J. R., Paulsen, J. S., Richardson, E. D., Springer, J. A., . . . Hines, M. E. (1990). The neuropathology of everyday life: The frequency of partial seizure symptoms among normals. *Neuropsychology, 4*, 65–86.

Ros, L. T. (2004). A case of "double" depression under outpatient treatment conditions. *World Journal of Biological Psychiatry, 5*, 161–163.

Rosenow, F., Wyllie, E., Kotagal, P., Mascha, E., Wolgamuth, B. R., & Hamer, H. (1998). Staring spells in children: Descriptive features distinguishing epileptic and nonepileptic events. *Journal of Pediatrics, 133*, 660–663.

Ruff, R. L., Ruff, S. S., & Wang, X. F. (2008). Headaches among Operation Iraqi Freedom/Operation Enduring Freedom veterans with mild traumatic brain injury associated with exposures to explosions. *Journal of Rehabilitation Research and Development, 45*, 941–952.

Sadler, R. M., & Rahey, S. (2004). Prescience as an aura of temporal lobe epilepsy. *Epilepsia, 45*, 982–984.

Sazgar, M., Carlen, P. L., & Wennberg, R. (2003). Panic attack semiology in right temporal lobe epilepsy. *Epileptic Disorders, 5*, 93–100.

Scherer, M. R., & Schubert, M. C. (2009). Traumatic brain injury and vestibular pathology as a comorbidity after blast exposure. *Physical Therapy, 89*, 980–992.

Sengoku, A., Toichi, M., & Murai, T. (1997). Dreamy states and psychoses in temporal lobe epilepsy: Mediating role of affect. *Psychiatry and Clinical Neuroscience, 51*, 23–26.

Setnik, L., & Bazarian, J. J. (2007). The characteristics of patients who do not seek medical treatment for traumatic brain injury. *Brain Injury, 21*, 1–9.

Shewmon, D. A., & Erwin, R. J. (1989). Transient impairment of visual perception induced by single interictal occipital spikes. *Journal of Clinical and Experimental Neuropsychology, 11*, 657–681.

Silvestri, R., & Bromfield, E. (2004). Recurrent nightmares and disorders of arousal in temporal lobe epilepsy. *Brain Research Bulletin, 63*, 369–376.

Sjaastad, O., Bakketeig, L. S., & Petersen, H. C. (2006). Migraine with aura: Visual disturbances and interrelationship with the pain phase. *Journal of Headache Pain, 7*, 127–135.

Smith, P. F., & Darlington, C. L. (2005). Drug treatments for subjective tinnitus: Serendipitous discovery versus rational drug design. *Current Opinion in Investigative Drugs, 6*, 712–716.

Smith Doody, R., Hrachovy, R. A., & Feher, E. P. (1992). Recurrent fluent aphasia associated with a seizure focus. *Brain & Language, 42*, 419–430.

Spitz, M. C. (1991). Panic disorder in seizure patients: A diagnostic pitfall. *Epilepsia, 32*, 33–38.

Stanford, M. S., Houston, R. J., & Baldridge, R. M. (2008). Comparison of impulsive and premeditated perpetrators of intimate partner violence. *Behavioral Science and Law, 26*, 709–722.

Stanford, M. S., Houston, R. J., Mathias, C. W., Villemarette-Pittman, N. R., Helfriz, L. E., & Conklin, S. M. (2003). Characterizing aggressive behavior. *Assessment, 10*, 183–190.

Stewart, J. T., & Bartucci, R. J. (1986). Posttraumatic stress disorder and partial complex seizures. *American Journal of Psychiatry, 143*, 113–114.

Striano, P., Zara, F., & Striano, S. (2010). Transient epileptic amnesia: A new epileptic syndrome in development? *Annals of Neurology, 67*, 416.

Sumer, M. M., Atik, L., Unal, A., Emre, U., & Atasoy, H. T. (2007). Frontal lobe epilepsy presented as ictal aggression. *Neurological Science, 28*, 48–51.

Syvertsen, M., Helde, G., Stovner, L. J., & Brodtkorb, E. (2007). Headaches add to the burden of epilepsy. *Journal of Headache Pain, 8,* 224–230.

Tay, S. Y., Ang, B. T., Lau, X. Y., Meyyappan, A., & Collinson, S. L. (2010). Chronic impairment of prospective memory after mild traumatic brain injury. *Journal of Neurotrauma, 27,* 77–83.

Taylor, D. C., & Lochery, M. (1987). Temporal lobe epilepsy: Origin and significance of simple and complex auras. *Journal of Neurology, Neurosurgery, and Psychiatry, 50,* 673–681.

Taylor, I., Scheffer, I. E., & Berkovic, S. F. (2003). Occipital epilepsies: Identification of specific and newly recognized syndromes. *Brain, 126,* 753–769.

Taylor, M. A. (1999). *Fundamentals of Clinical Neuropsychiatry.* New York, NY: Oxford University Press.

Theeler, B. J., & Erickson, J. C. (2009). Mild head trauma and chronic headaches in returning US soldiers. *Headache, 49,* 529–534.

Thijs, R. D., Bloem, B. R., & van Dijk, J. G. Falls, faints, fits and funny turns. *Journal of Neurology, 256,* 155–167.

Tombini, M., Koch, G., Placidi, F., Sancesario, G., Marciani, M. G., & Bernardi, G. (2005). Temporal lobe epileptic activity mimicking dementia: A case report. *European Journal of Neurology, 12,* 805–806.

Trebuchon-Da Fonseca, A., Guedj, E., Alario, F. X., Laguitton, V., Mundler, O., Chauvel, P., & Liegeois-Chauvel, C. (2009). Brain regions underlying word finding difficulties in temporal lobe epilepsy. *Brain, 132,* 2772–2784.

Treiman, D. M. (1991). Psychobiology of ictal aggression. *Advances in Neurology, 55,* 341–356.

Tuxhorn, I. E. (2005). Somatosensory auras in focal epilepsy: A clinical, video EEG, and MRI study. *Seizure, 14,* 262–268.

Van Paesschen, W., King, M. D., Duncan, J. S., & Connelly, A. (2001). The amygdala and temporal lobe simple partial seizures: A prospective and quantitative MRI study. *Epilepsia, 42,* 857–862.

Weiss, G. M., & Spiegel, D. R. (2008). Transient amnestic syndrome in the setting of recurrent partial elementary seizures. *Journal of Neuropsychiatry and Clinical Neuroscience, 20,* 115–116.

Weissman, D. H., Roberts, K. C., Visscher, K. M., & Woldorff, M. G. (2006). The neural bases of momentary lapses in attention. *Nature Neuroscience, 9,* 971–978.

Wild, E. (2005). Déjà vu in neurology. *Journal of Neurology, 252,* 1–7.

Williams, D. (1956). The structure of emotions reflected in epileptic experiences. *Brain, 79,* 29–67.

Yang, C. C., Hua, M. S., Tu, Y. K., & Huang, S. J. (2009). Early clinical characteristics of patients with persistent post-concussion symptoms: a prospective study. *Brain Injury, 23,* 299–306.

Yu, L., & Blumenfeld, H. (2009). Theories of impaired consciousness in epilepsy. *Annals of the New York Academy of Science, 1157,* 48–60.

Zijlmans, M., van Eijsden, P., Ferier, C. H., Kho, K. H., van Rijen, P. C., Leijten, F. S. (2009). Illusory shadow person causing paradoxical gaze deviations during temporal lobe seizures. *Journal of Neurology, Neurosurgery, & Psychiatry, 80,* 686–688.

APPENDIX

II

Making the Diagnosis of MIND in Adult Patients

Virtually all DSM-IV-TR psychiatric diagnoses are based upon self-report data (e.g., "I feel depressed"), observations of significant others in the patient's environment (e.g., "He appeared to be talking with someone even though no one is in the room with him."), and judgments on the part of a trained diagnostician (e.g., "The patient meets DSM-IV-R criteria for the diagnosis of PTSD").The procedures for diagnosing MIND to be described in this chapter also rely on self-report data, observational data, and clinical judgment. However, one difference between making the proposed diagnosis of MIND and making most DSM-IV-TR diagnoses is that we have chosen to link diagnosis of MIND to a particular assessment procedure: the Iowa Interview, the content of which was discussed extensively in Technical Appendix I. To a certain extent, this decision makes the proposed diagnosis of MIND an *operational diagnosis* because it is tied to the operations of administering, scoring, and interpreting the results of the Iowa Interview in light of what is known about the patient.

However, interviewing for symptoms of MIND is based largely on phenomenology, observational data from others, and clinical judgments made by the interviewer. In this sense, making the proposed diagnosis is not unlike the processes care providers use for making DSM-IV-TR-type diagnoses.

The Iowa Interview was developed specifically to assess for episodic or intermittent symptoms following mild-to-moderate TBI due to blunt-force trauma (Roberts et al., 1990; Roberts, 1999).The decision to use a structured interview format later was supported by research indicating that asking patients to simply fill out questionnaires regarding post-concussive symptoms may lead to symptom over-endorsement (Iverson, Brooks, Ashton, & Lange, 2010). In the clinical setting, the Iowa Interview is administered only after the patients (and any collateral informants) have been interviewed in an open-ended (nonstructured) fashion to determine their spontaneous complaints (cf., Nolin, Villemure, & Heroux, 2006).

The interview consists of a total of 40 items (refer to Table I–1). All but one item is rated for estimated *frequency of occurrence* on a 7-point scale (0 = *never or not in the past year*, 1 = *two or three times in the past year*, 2 = *at least once a month*, 3 = *at least once a week*, 4 = *several times a week*, 5 = *once a day*, 6 = *more than once a day*). (Only the "Mental Decline" item (31) is rated on a dichotomous No = 0, Yes = 6 *basis*.) In contrast to the Iowa Interview, virtually all checklists for postconcussive symptoms (e.g., the Rivermead) require the patient to rate the severity of each PCS symptom. After pilot studies, we decided that asking the patient to estimate frequency of occurrence for each symptom on the Iowa Interview was a better format than asking the patient to estimate the *severity* of each symptom or using a dichotomous "Yes/No" format for all items (e.g., Elgmark Andersson, Emanuelson, Olsson, Stalhammer, & Starmark, 2006).

The item content of the current version of Iowa Interview was published in Roberts (1999) as the Iowa Interview for Partial Seizure-like Symptoms and, thus, has been in the public domain for more than a decade. Normative data for total score, based upon the interview responses of 115 normal, young adults without history of head trauma, is presented in Table II–1. [In hindsight, the authors of the interview would not have used the words "partial seizure-like" when referring to symptoms, preferring neutral language such as "intermittent" or "episodic" symptoms; however, an earlier version of the interview was first published in 1990, and the authors of that article followed Tucker, Price, Johnson, and McAllister (1986) in assuming that such symptoms reflected underlying electrical instability similar to that associated with conventional complex partial seizures. Currently, it seems clear that most MIND patients lack at least three key features of conventional complex partial seizure disorders: a stereotyped course of spells, motor automatisms, and complete alteration of consciousness.]

Table II-1. Normative Data for the 40-Item Version of the Iowa Interview (IIPSS) for Adults

Total Score	n	Percentile
>70	1	—
60–69	2	99th
50–59	4	97th
40–49	9	94th
30–39	10	87th
20–29	27	77th
10–19	38	54th
0–9	24	21st

From: Roberts, R. J. (1999). Epilepsy Spectrum Disorder in the context of mild traumatic brain injury. In N. R. Varney & R. J. Roberts (Eds.), *The evaluation and treatment of mild traumatic brain injury* (pp. 409–447). Mahwah, NJ: Lawrence Erlbaum.

The total score on the interview is calculated by summing the numerical responses to all 40 items. The 95th percentile cutoff for the total score is 50 for young adults. The 90th percentile cutoff is a total score of 40. The form for the Iowa Interview published in Roberts (1999) also includes the 90th percentile cutoffs for each item individually, so that the interviewer has some guidance as to which responses to *individual items* are frequent enough to warrant further clinical inquiry.

The proposed research diagnostic criteria for making the diagnosis of MIND in the context of blunt force TBI in adults are presented in Table II–2. Because we are proposing that MIND is likely to be a distinctive subtype of Persistent Postconcussional Disorder following blunt-force head trauma, Criterion A specifies

Table II-2. Proposed Research Diagnostic Criteria for a MIND Subtype of PPCS Following Blunt-Force Head Trauma in Adults

A. Patient meets DSM-IV-R criteria for Post-concussional Disorder with significant symptoms persisting for at least six months following an instance of concussion or mild TBI.

B. The patient obtains a total score of 50 or greater (at or above the 95th percentile of the healthy standardization group: $N = 115$) on the Iowa Interview for partial seizure-like symptoms. The patient endorses at least one episodic symptom with clinically significant frequency (i.e., at or above the 90th percentile of a normal standardization sample) in *each* of the following domains of episodic symptoms: psycho-sensory, cognitive, and affective.

C. The elevated number of intermittent symptoms does not appear to be reasonably attributable to marked dissociative processes associated with a history of severe child abuse or with extreme emotional traumatization in adult life.

D. The patient has never sustained any severe febrile illness in adulthood with fever of 105°F or higher; does not have clinically significant exposure to toxic chemicals; has never experienced significant hypoxia (e.g., CO poisoning, cardiac resuscitation, near-drowning);

Table II–2. *continued*

has never experienced an instance of blast exposure in military or civilian life; does not manifest untreated sleep apnea.

E. In between episodic or transitory symptoms, interpersonal rapport and social functioning appear to be within relatively broad normal limits in that continuous psychosis is absent.

F. The patient's symptoms do not appear to reflect malingering.

Frequently *associated* (but nonessential) *features* include the following:

(1) possible deficits with executive function (particularly if the patient is anosmic or hyposmic on actual testing); (2) possible history of multiple instances of blunt-force trauma; (3) chronic dysphoria with possible suicidal ideation (meeting DSM-IV criteria for major depression does note rule out making the MIND diagnosis); (4) there may be some overlap with Intermittent Explosive Disorder, and hostile-aggressive outbursts tend to be irritable (or impulsive) rather than premeditated (or instrumental)—often with genuine remorse or incomprehension spontaneously expressed; (5) roughly 40% of MIND patients have at least mild EEG abnormalities, but only 10–15% have clearly epileptiform findings; (6) largely negative neurological exam and structural neuro-imaging studies; (7) 60–70% chance of defective Dichotic Word Listening Performance in the context of normal hearing, as assessed by pure-tone audiometry; (8) a tendency to produce grossly elevated MMPI-2 profiles, with 6 to 8 of 10 clinical scales at T-score of 65 or higher; (9) poor past response to psychotropic medications that tend to lower seizure threshold (e.g., phenothiazines, lithium, buproprion), with limited positive responses to SSRIs and/or cognitive therapies; (10) risk for misuse of substances that increase seizure-threshold (e.g., alcohol, benzodiazepines); (11) problems with educational or vocational status due to transitory cognitive lapses; (12) increased risk for marital/family arguments revolving around unrecalled or incorrectly recalled conversations.

that the patient must meet the DSM-IV-R criteria for Postconcus-sional Disorder following blunt-force or acceleration-deceleration head trauma and that significant impairment still persists for at least 6 months following the acute trauma. The requirement of dysfunction that persists for 6 months may seem overly conservative. However, we generally have chosen to be conservative because of the controversial nature of the debate over PPCS and mild TBI.

Criterion B requires a total score of 50 or more on the Iowa Interview. In selecting this rather stringent cutoff, we have once again chosen to be conservative. In actual clinical practice, it is likely that some patients with total scores in the range between 40 and 49 (i.e., above the 90th percentile) also may respond well to clinical trial of mood stabilizers with anticonvulsant properties.

Criterion C requires that a given patient must produce a clinically significant score (i.e., at or above the 90th percentile of the standardization group) on one of the items in each of the psychosensory, cognitive, and affective item clusters. Inclusion of this criterion was designed to ensure that a given patient would manifest at least a minimal breadth of intermittent symptoms in daily functioning.

Criterion D was included because some patients with severely dissociative pathology appear to generate relatively high scores on a dissociative basis that is unlikely to be due to head trauma (Bob, Susta, Paviat, Hynek, & Raboch, 2005; Roca & Freeman, 2002). Ross (1994) has published an extensive case study of a highly dissociative patient who reported experiencing multiple intermittent symptoms in the context of a history of severe, psychological traumatization. For research purposes, a patient who appears to be highly dissociative and who generates a high score on the Iowa Interview probably should be excluded from a formal treatment study unless a clear link is described between an instance of head trauma and the onset of intermittent symptoms.

However, the treating clinician is in a rather difficult situation when a patient has a well-documented history of severe dissociation *and* a well-documented history of head trauma (Cantagallo, Grassi, & Della Sala, 1999; Mula et al., 2006; Sulloway &

White, 1997; Tucker, 1998). Histories of occult head trauma may occur in connection with other forms of child abuse and neglect (Chiesa & Duhaime, 2009; Christian & Block, 2009; Rubin, Christian, Bilaniuk, Zazyczny, & Durbin, 2003) and in the context of spousal abuse (Banks, 2007; Sheridan & Nash, 2007). Furthermore, early childhood abuse may be associated with experiencing of more intermittent symptoms even in the absence of head trauma (Teicher, Glod, Surrey, & Swett, 1993). As discussed in earlier chapters on blast exposure, military service in a combat zone frequently is associated with both psychological trauma and increased risk of head trauma or blast exposure (Taneilian & Jaycox, 2008). Additionally complicating matters is the fact that dissociative disorders often are diagnosed based largely upon the "exclusion of organic pathology" rather than clear inclusion criteria, as Brown & Trimble (2000) have pointed out. Until additional research findings provide some sort of rational basis for sorting out these complexities, assessing Criterion D in diagnosing MIND is likely to depend largely upon the judgment of the clinician making the assessment.

The intention behind including Criterion E was to exclude potential causes for MIND symptomatology other than blunt-force and acceleration-deceleration forms of head trauma for research purposes. We have observed that severe febrile illnesses in adulthood, episodes of hypoxia, exposures to some neuro-toxins, and exposure to blast concussion can all produce clinically elevated scores on the Iowa Interview. Clinically, the intermittent symptoms of patients with other etiologies may well respond to treatment with mood stabilizers (e.g., Roberts, 2008); however, the decision to rule out other potential etiologies was once again made to err on the side of being conservative for the purposes of research. The exclusion of patients with untreated sleep apnea syndromes reflects the high incidence of sleep-disordered breathing in the American veteran population (Ocasio-Tascon, Alicea-Colon, Torres-Palacios, & Rodriguez-Clintron, 2006).

Criterion F is based upon the observations of other experts (especially Tucker et al., 1986, and Taylor, 1999), as well as our own. Although Tucker et al. initially used the term "atypical psychosis" as one of the descriptors for MIND-like patients, he was clear that, in between intermittent spells, his patients behaved in a relatively sociable, nonpsychotic fashion (i.e., they did not constantly hallucinate, conversation was broadly normal). Two caveats deserve comment here. First, if a given patient has sustained damage to, or dysfunction, in the prefrontal region of the brain due to head trauma, then the patient may manifest psychosocial deficits that commonly appear following prefrontal damage (Anderson, Barrash, Bechara, & Tranel, 2006; Wood, 2009). The effects of such damage can occur even in the absence of clear cognitive deficits on most structured neuropsychological tests. Second, just as a given medical patient may develop two unrelated medical diseases (diabetes and COPD, for example), a given patient with pre-existing psychiatric disorder (e.g., schizophrenia, PTSD, antisocial personality disorder) may sustain an instance of blunt-force head trauma and subsequently develop symptoms of PPCS and MIND. Put another way, symptoms of other comorbid neuropsychiatric disorders can make it more difficult for a clinician to make a clean diagnosis of MIND.

The focus of Criterion G, the absence of malingering, reflects the current debate regarding mild TBI in general. A computer literature search on the intersection of the terms "traumatic brain injury and malingering" identified 211 separate articles, of which 191 were published since 1990. In contrast, a computer literature search on "major depression and malingering" produced only 49 articles in total, of which 41 were published since 1990. Similarly, the corresponding figures for "schizophrenia and malingering" were 62 and 38, respectively. Clearly, many neuropsychological researchers have devoted a great deal of attention to studying malingering in the context of a reported history of head trauma following Faust and Ziskind's (1988) attack on the adequacy of courtroom testimony from expert witnesses in neuropsychology.

One of the most important things to realize is that the base rate of true "malingering" is likely to depend in large part upon the nature of one's clinical practice (Ruff, 2009). Although it has become a characteristic of practice for many neuropsychologists to include at least one formal test for "malingering" or "poor effort" in forensic exams, the outcomes from such tasks need to be considered in the broad context of what is known about the patient. A comprehensive resource on the assessment of malingering, instruments to assess malingering, and "effort tests" has been edited by Larrabee (2007).

The paragraph at the bottom of Table II–2 lists associated, but nonessential, clinical features of patients who receive the MIND diagnosis. The interested reader is referred to R. J. Roberts (1999, Chapter 11, pp. 409–447) for additional details and references supporting the clinical observations at the bottom of the table.

References

Anderson, S. W., Barrash, J., Bechara, A., & Tranel, D. (2006). Impairments of emotion and real-world complex behavior following childhood- or adult-onset damage to ventromedial prefrontal cortex. *Journal of the International Neuropsychological Society, 12,* 224–235.

Banks, M. E. (2007). Overlooked but critical: Traumatic brain injury as a consequence of interpersonal violence. *Trauma, Violence, and Abuse, 8,* 290–298.

Bob, P., Susta, M., Pavlat, J., Hynek, K., & Raboch, J. (2005). Depression, traumatic dissociation and epileptic-like phenomena. *Neurology and Endocrinology Letters, 26,* 321–325.

Brown, R. J., & Trimble, M. R. (2000). Dissociative psychopathology, non-epileptic seizures, and neurology. *Journal of Neurology, Neurosurgery, and Psychiatry, 69,* 285–289.

Cantagallo, A., Grassi, L., & Della Sala, S. (1999). Dissociative disorder after traumatic brain injury. *Brain Injury, 13,* 219–228.

Chiesa, A., & Duhaime, A. C. (2009). Abusive head trauma. *Pediatric Clinics of North America, 56,* 317–331.

Christian, C. W., & Block, R. (2009). Committee on Child Abuse and Neglect; American Academy of Pediatrics. *Pediatrics, 123,* 1409–1411.

Elgmark Anderrson, E., Emanuelson, I., Olsson, M., Stalhammar, D., & Starmark, J. E. (2006). The new Swedish Post-Concussion

Symptoms questionnaire: A measure of symptoms after mild traumatic brain injury and its concurrent validity and inter-rater reliability. *Journal of Rehabilitation Medicine, 38,* 26–31.

Faust, D., & Ziskind, J. (1988). The expert witness in psychology and psychiatry. *Science, 241,* 31–35.

Iverson, G. L., Brooks, B. L., Ashton, V. L., & Lange, R. T. (2010). Interview versus questionnaire symptom reporting in people with the postconcussion syndrome. *Journal of Head Trauma Rehabilitation, 25,* 23–30.

Larrabee, G. J. (2007). *Assessment of malingered neuropsychological deficits.* New York, NY: Oxford University Press.

Mula, M., Cavanna, A., Collimedaglia, L., Barbagi, D., Magli, E., & Monaco, F. (2006). The role of aura in psychopathology and dissociative experiences in epilepsy. *Journal of Neuropsychiatry and Clinical Neuroscience, 18,* 536–542.

Nolin P., Villemure, R., & Theroux, L. (2006). Determining long-term symptoms following mild traumatic brain injury: Method of interview affects self-report. *Brain Injury, 20,* 1147–1154.

Ocasio-Tascon, M. E., Alicea-Colon, E., Torres-Palacious, A., & Rodriguez-Cintron, W. (2006). The veteran population: One at high risk for sleep-disordered breathing. *Sleep and Breathing, 10,* 70–75.

Roberts, R. J. (2008, December–January). Impact on the brain. *Scientific American Mind,* 50–57.

Roberts, R. J. (1999). Epilepsy Spectrum Disorder in the context of mild traumatic brain injury. In N. R. Varney & R. J. Roberts (Eds.), *The evaluation and treatment of mild traumatic brain injury* (pp. 409–447). Mahwah, NJ: Lawrence Erlbaum.

Roberts, R. J., Varney, N. R., Hulbert, J. R., Paulsen, J. S., Richard-son, E. D., Springer, J. A., . . . Hines, M.E. (1990). The neu-ropathology of everyday life: The frequency of partial seizure symptoms among normals. *Neuropsychology, 4,* 65–86.

Roca, V., & Freeman, T. W. (2002). Psychosensory symptoms in combat veterans with posttraumatic stress disorder. *Journal of Neuropsychiatry and Clinical Neuroscience, 14,* 185–189.

Ross, C. (1994). *The Osiris Complex.* Toronto, Canada: University of Toronto Press.

Rubin, D. M., Christian, C. W., Bilaniuk, L. T., Zazyczny, K. A., & Durbin, D. R., (2003). Occult head injury in high-risk abused children. *Pediatrics, 151*, 1382–1386.

Ruff, R. (2009). Best practice guidelines for forensic neuropsychological examinations of patients with traumatic brain injury. *Journal of Head Trauma Rehabilitation, 24*, 131–140.

Salloway, S., & White, J. (1997). Paroxysmal limbic disorders in neuropsychiatry. *Journal of Neuropsychiatry and Clinical Neuroscience, 9*, 403–419.

Sheridan, D. J., & Nash, K. R. (2007). Acute injury patterns of intimate partner violence victims. *Trauma, Violence, and Abuse, 8*, 281–289.

Tanielian, T., & Jaycox, L. H. (2008). *The invisible wounds of war.* Santa Monica, CA: Rand Corporation.

Taylor, M. A. (1999). *Fundamentals of Clinical Neuropsychiatry.* New York, NY: Oxford University Press.

Teicher, M. H., Glod, C. A., Surrey, J., Swett, C., Jr. (1993). Early childhood abuse and limbic system ratings in adult psychiatric outpatients. *Journal of Neuropsychiatry and Clinical Neuroscience, 5*, 301–306.

Tucker, G. J. (1998). Seizure disorders presenting with psychiatric symptomatology. *Psychiatry Clinics of North America, 21*, 625–635.

Tucker, G. J., Price, T. R. P., Johnson, V. B., & McAllister, T. (1986). Phenomenology of temporal lobe dysfunction: A link to atypical psychosis—a series of cases. *Journal of Nervous and Mental Disease, 174*, 348–356.

Wood, R. L. (2009). The scientist-practitioner model: How do advances in clinical and cognitive neuroscience affect neuropsychology in the courtroom. *Journal of Head Trauma Rehabilitation, 24*, 88–99.

Index

Bold denotes nontext material.